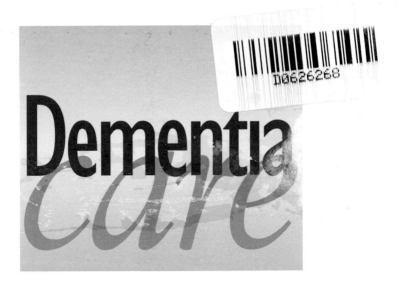

A HANDBOOK FOR RESIDENTIAL AND DAY CARE

Alan Chapman, Alan Jacques and Mary Marshall

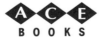

ACE
BOOKS

© 1994 Alan Chapman, Alan Jacques and Mary Marshall
Published by Age Concern England
1268 London Road
London SW16 4ER

Editor Gillian Clarke
Production Marion Peat
Design and typesetting Eugenie Dodd
Copy preparation Vinnette Marshall
Printed and bound in Great Britain by Bell & Bain Ltd, Glasgow

A catalogue record for this book is available from the British Library.

ISBN 0–86242–128–4

Contents

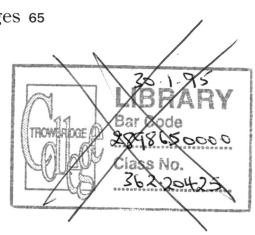

About the Authors

Alan Chapman is the Training Officer at the Dementia Services Development Centre at the University of Stirling. He previously worked as a Staff Development Officer (Elderly Care) in a local authority social services department.

Dr Alan Jacques is a consultant in old age psychiatry at the Royal Victoria Hospital, Edinburgh. He is Vice-chairman of Alzheimer Scotland – Action on Dementia, and the author of *Understanding Dementia*.

Professor Mary Marshall is the Director of the Dementia Services Development Centre at the University of Stirling. She was previously Director of Age Concern Scotland.

Acknowledgements

The authors thank Val Good, Staff Officer, East Sussex County Council, Lewes, and Sandra James, Sessional Training Officer, Dementia Services Development Centre, Stirling, for assistance with the text.

They are also grateful to Philip Chan, Community Relations Officer, Community Relations Council, Edinburgh, for his comments on the case study of Mr Ho; and to Rahat Syyed, Senior Care Worker with the Dixon Community Ethnic Elderly Project, Glasgow, for her comments on the case study of Mrs Begum.

Introduction

WHY A DEMENTIA GUIDE?

Working in a nursing or residential Home or a day care centre is a complex mix of roles and responsibilities. You have to provide consistent and high quality care to everyone – whether they are residents or day care clients – remembering always that they are individuals with different backgrounds and varying needs.

Providing continuity of care to people with dementia is no easy matter. The main aim of this guide is to stress that individuals should be respected and valued for their life experience and life history because their pathway through the illness is so bound up in their past. Although deficits will be very obvious, it is essential that you focus on whatever ability remains. Kitwood and Bredin in their book, *Person to Person*, suggest that maintaining good relationships with staff and other residents or day care clients is a vital part of how the person with dementia copes with the illness.

It is a basic assumption of this book that the quality of life for people with dementia and their carers should be at the highest possible level. The King's Fund has drawn up the following list of principles that are important in providing care and should be considered by all staff groups.

People with dementia have the same human value as anyone else, irrespective of their degree of disability or independence

People who do not work and people who have serious disabilities risk being undervalued in our society; women, too, are often undervalued. Many people with dementia fall into all three of these categories, and so they are at risk on all three counts. Our expectations about quality of life for people with dementia must not be allowed to fall below the standards of other members of the community. We should be concerned not just with meeting minimum standards but also with demonstrating positively the value and importance of older people and people with dementia.

People with dementia have the same varied human needs as anyone else

This means not only basic needs for food, warmth, shelter and protection from physical hurt, but also for affection, companionship and opportunities to take part in worthwhile activities. People with dementia are entitled to share in the whole range of life's experiences, alongside other citizens in the mainstream of society. Only when they live as others do can people with dementia be accepted as having equal value. Only by living as others do will they have access to the same range of human contacts and resources. To achieve that objective for people with severe dementia and to help them enjoy some of the benefits of community life will require a high level of long-term support, professional skill, imagination and resources.

People with dementia have the same rights as other citizens

People with dementia are often denied opportunities and resources to which they have a right. In many cases, this is because they are unable to assert their just demands. It is the duty of those who serve them to find ways to claim on their behalf and to preserve their rights jealously. When formal steps are taken to change the legal status of an individual, the safeguards and access to representation should be the highest standard expected by other citizens.

Every person with dementia is an individual

People with dementia, like anyone else, have the right to behave as individuals, within the limits of the law, and to be seen as individuals with their own preferences, abilities and needs.

One part of 'individuality' is being helped in ways that are personally tailored to you. A second part is making sure that your individual history and past life are not lost and forgotten by those around you. Individuality means having continuity between your past, your present and your future.

People with dementia have the right to forms of support that do not exploit family and friends

It is the informal support of families, friends and neighbours that provides the major proportion of help for people with dementia. These carers have the right to expect a normal quality of life without being exposed to stress and exhaustion. Those who provide services have a duty to ensure that they actively recognise and support the work carried out by carers.

Do remember that there will be situations in which the needs and wishes of the older person conflict with those of their relatives. Professional carers should be concerned that the rights of both parties are safeguarded.

Using the book

This book discusses all the areas associated with providing care to people with dementia. It draws on the results of current research and the authors' work experiences with managers, staff and people with dementia and their carers.

The book has been written for managers and care staff, to help you think about the caring that goes on in your Home or day centre. At the end of each chapter there are suggested training exercises, which are to encourage self-study. They are intended to prompt your thinking about what you have read. If you seriously attempt these you will be able to use this guide as a resource to improving the quality of the care you provide. Ideally, write your ideas down in a notebook if you are doing these questions on your own. You should then share your ideas with other staff.

In Appendix 1 are model answers to the questions posed. They are not intended to be the ideal but we think that, if followed, they could lead to good practice.

Typical residents and day care clients are introduced below – Mrs Florence Amble, Mrs Fatima Begum, Mr Ho Ming, Miss Amy Peacock and Mr John Hastie – whose stories are based on real-life situations. Throughout the book, their experiences are described to illustrate certain points.

Time

Managers and care staff are busy people, so the idea of spending a lot of time at one go reading this book may be off-putting. We suggest that you plan to read this guide over a period of a few weeks, spending at least 15 minutes at a time on each chapter – perhaps making brief notes as you read. Alternatively, you may like to use part of a staff meeting to discuss the questions raised.

Meet Mrs Amble, Mr Ho, Mrs Begum, Mr Hastie and Miss Peacock

Mrs Florence Amble is 85 years of age. Since the death of her husband 18 months ago she has lived alone, with support from her neighbours. She has attended the local day hospital for day care during the past six months, because she has developed symptoms of dementia.

Mrs Amble has no close relatives and is heavily dependent on the support of her home care assistant, Jean, who lives in the next street. Neighbours are increasingly concerned because she often leaves the gas cooker turned on and not lit, or lit and burning her pots. She also smokes in bed and the fire brigade have been called to the house twice in the last month. Jean has reported that Mrs Amble is becoming increasingly muddled and has taken to getting up during the night and wandering outside her house, looking for her son.

The social worker has been unable to contact any next of kin but has decided that Mrs Amble should be admitted to your Home.

Mr Ho Ming is 61 years of age. He has lived for the past 40 years in London, having emigrated from Hong Kong. He set up a take-away business which over the years has prospered and he now owns a restaurant. His British-born wife and three sons are all involved in the businesses. Mr Ho has always worked long hours in the restaurant or take-away and did the tasks from cooking and preparing the food and meals to serving the meals or cleaning the premises.

Lately, since he suffered a couple of strokes, his family feel that he has become lethargic, increasingly confused and withdrawn, and he is now communicating only in a Cantonese dialect. One son has had to act as a sitter but, because of the pressure of work and family ties, the family have agreed that Mr Ho would be better off in a Home. They all work very long hours and the alternative is locking Mr Ho into the house while they are at work.

The GP has telephoned your Home, asking if you could admit Mr Ho immediately.

Mrs Fatima Begum is a devout Muslim woman originally from a village in Northern Pakistan. She moved into the Home two years ago after having a stroke which left her physically very disabled. She is now 74 years of age.

She came to the UK twenty years ago to set up a grocery store with her husband and family. Her husband died ten years ago. The family later found that they were unable to look after her and run the shop so they requested her admission.

Mrs Begum is very settled in the Home. With the help of the local mosque the staff are able to assist Mrs Begum with the timing of her wadoo (preparation for prayer) and prayers in the quiet place she has chosen. Staff have also arranged for supplies of halal food with the help of her family. Mrs Begum is gaining a great deal of pleasure from the company of a new care assistant, Mrs Ali. They can talk Urdu together and both enjoy reading the Koran.

As part of a Care in the Community strategy, the Home has begun to offer day care, and has employed an outreach worker and an activities organiser. Mr Hastie and Miss Peacock are the first two individuals to attend day care. The Home intends to create a special day care lounge/dining area but at present Mr Hastie and Miss Peacock sit in the residents' lounge.

Mr John Hastie, a keen golfer, worked as a foreman for a firm of builders for 25 years. He retired three years ago at the age of 65. He lives with his wife in a block of flats. Six months ago he suffered a stroke, which has caused a degree of confusion and mild paralysis of his left side. The paralysis affects his walking – he has a definite limp/shuffle of his left foot. He slurs his words when talking and he has problems with chewing food.

Mr Hastie attends day care in the Home for two days a week, from 10.00 am to 2.00 pm; a minibus picks him up from home in the morning and returns him in the afternoon. This gives his wife respite. She shows signs of frustration and anger at Mr Hastie's behaviour: he shouts at her but communicates little and is not interested in the television – he wants to lie in bed all day.

Day care provides activities that can help with his confusion and also help him to regain some skills in caring for himself.

Mr Hastie seems to be quite happy most of the time in day care. He enjoys the activities but believes that the minibus is taking him to work. He often walks around the Home banging walls and shouting that the wall needs to be rebuilt, and he is continually following staff around.

Miss Amy Peacock is a retired sister of a children's ward in a hospital, where she worked for 35 years. She cared for her mother, who died last year at the age of 98. Miss Peacock had taken early retirement at 60, two years ago, to care for her mother.

Since the death of her mother, Miss Peacock has become extremely disorientated and confused. She keeps walking out of her house looking for her mother – she thinks that her mother has gone on holiday and left her behind. She knocks on neighbours' doors in the middle of the night.

Miss Peacock refuses to allow the home care assistant into the house but likes the 'young lady' (the outreach worker) who calls and brings her out of the house. At day care, she sits in the lounge, retelling stories of what she did as a sister but she becomes agitated at any mention of her mother.

Miss Peacock is very prim and proper, and she complains about ineffective staff.

1 Caring for the Individual

In this chapter we will consider what dementia is and what it is not, how it affects individuals and what we can do to help.

DEMENTIA IS MORE THAN FORGETTING

Things around us change over time and so do we. When we look at other people, particularly groups of other people, we see that children do more than grow bigger when becoming adolescent; they change. Adolescents 'mature' into young adults who become more settled in middle age. 'Old age' is a time of life that few admit they have actually reached, even when given the hint by the issue of a bus pass and pension. The saying 'you're only as old as you feel' is true for many.

Some changes do come with growing older:

- physical appearance;
- skin texture;
- muscle strength;
- stamina and nimbleness;
- bones and joints;
- eyesight;
- hearing.

All these become less sound than they were. Illnesses, old and new, may accumulate and mean that we need to take medicines to keep reasonably well.

It is important to remember, though, that not all change is inevitable. What makes older people seem different is:

- their way of thinking;
- their way of living;
- their social relationships with others.

People who enter retirement in their sixties these days are generally much fitter than people of the same age in the 1930s and 1940s.

DEMENTIA: HOW COMMON IS IT?

Dementia as an illness is different from normal ageing. It is a terminal illness which, over time, leads to great changes in the person.

It is rare in anyone younger than 60 years of age. Before that age, it is more likely to be due to physical problems such as injuries to the head or a brain tumour.

It becomes increasingly common among very old people. Between the ages of 60 years and 79 years, approximately 4 per cent (1 in 25) of people will show symptoms of dementia. This figure increases to 15 per cent (1 in 6) for those aged over 80 years.

WHAT IS DEMENTIA?

The symptoms of dementia usually develop slowly and it may be difficult to pinpoint when the change began. Most families will have noticed mild forgetfulness, or mixing up days and times, or getting muddled with bills or tablets, as the first hint that something was wrong, though only later will they realise the significance of these changes. Families often search their memories for a point when their relative's dementia began, but this is not necessarily the 'onset time'.

Sometimes the dementia begins suddenly, after the person has been temporarily confused by a physical illness. Often families will say: 'She's never been the same since Dad died', or 'They should never have moved', dating the onset to change of social circumstances, which again may have been temporarily confusing.

Dementia gradually affects the ability of the person to:

- remember things for more than a few seconds;
- make sense of the world around them;
- cope with the tasks of daily living;
- express their feelings;
- take initiatives or plan;
- think clearly and solve problems;
- cope with an over-stimulating environment;
- behave in the normal ways they have learned during their lives.

All these changes are directly due to the damage to nerve cells and the messages they pass, which happen in all the different illnesses that cause dementia.

Alzheimer's disease

Two out of three people who develop dementia are suffering from dementia of the Alzheimer type (DAT), sometimes called Alzheimer's disease. Research has shown that Alzheimer's dementia is caused by damage to certain types of nerve cell in the brain. The brain works by sending countless chemical messages between billions of microscopic nerve cells. There are many different sorts of these cells and only certain types are involved in Alzheimer's, mainly those where the messages to other cells are passed by a chemical called acetylcholine.

Scientists are beginning to understand why these particular nerve cells are damaged. For some years it was thought that aluminium played a part, but now this seems less likely. It seems more likely that some chemical within the brain, perhaps even a chemical that normally helps the brain to keep healthy, becomes poisonous (toxic) to the nerve cells, and so they do not function properly and may even die. A small number of younger people with Alzheimer's dementia develop it as a hereditary condition (the vast majority of cases are not hereditary), and many people who have Down's syndrome unfortunately develop Alzheimer's in middle age. These genetic causes are helping research workers to find what the toxic chemical is and how the damage is done.

In the meantime, treatments have been developed which, in the early stages of dementia, may reduce the effects of the damage to nerve cells and so give sufferers some months of a better life, before the damage becomes too severe. A lot more research will have to be done before there is a true cure that stops the damage happening in the first place. What we do know now is that Alzheimer's is no respecter of persons. It can happen to anyone from any walk of life. In fact, the older we get the greater the risk that we might develop Alzheimer's disease.

Vascular dementia

Up to one-fifth of people with dementia have what is called a vascular dementia; that is, they have diseases of the blood vessels that feed the brain. These people may have general arteriosclerosis (also called hardening of the arteries) with other diseases of their circulation such as heart disease or high blood pressure. One of the commonest types of vascular dementia is called multi-infarct dementia. In this the person suffers a series of small strokes. Men are more likely to be affected than women, and it tends to affect people at a slightly younger age.

Multi-infarct dementia may start suddenly, and sometimes the small strokes lead to:

- sudden deterioration in the person's mental condition, unlike the very steady decline of Alzheimer's disease;
- periods of more severe confusion or obvious physical effects which can last for anything from a few minutes to a few weeks;
- speech difficulties or paralysis.

Things may then be unchanged for a while or even get a little better before the disease continues its downhill course. More often, the progress of a vascular dementia is steadily downhill like Alzheimer's disease, and it can be very difficult to tell them apart. In the not-too-distant future we may be able to prevent the strokes that cause multi-infarct dementia, but at present the main effort is in ensuring that people lead healthy lives and so prevent damage to their blood vessels, and that blood pressure and heart problems are properly treated.

Other types of dementia

About 15 per cent of people with dementia are either suffering from dementia caused by Parkinson's disease, with the characteristic tremor and shuffling walk, or have an illness related to Parkinson's disease (called Lewy body dementia) in which they do not get the usual physical changes of parkinsonism but only the dementia. Again it is often difficult to tell the difference between this dementia and Alzheimer's or vascular dementia, even though it is caused by a completely different illness. In some cases Lewy body dementia follows a very different course, with many spells of confusion, a lot of hallucinations and a rapid decline to death. Unfortunately, the usual treatments for Parkinson's disease do not help in either of these two types of dementia.

The other 5 per cent of people with dementia will be suffering from one of the many rarer illnesses that can cause gradually increasing damage to the brain and result in a gradual mental decline. The list of these rarer causes includes alcohol (this dementia sometimes improves if the person stops drinking), hydrocephalus (water on the brain) as a result of past head injuries (which may be treated), rare virus conditions such as Creutzfeldt–Jakob disease, AIDS, and some very treatable medical conditions such as thyroid disorder.

In general, however, most dementia either is caused by Alzheimer's disease or is vascular. Sadly, there is no cure at present for either condition. Whatever the cause, the symptoms and the general course of dementia are roughly the same – starting from that person's normal, they gradually decline mentally till their death.

WHAT DEMENTIA IS NOT

It is important to know that having a poor memory for certain things, such as names, is not a sign of dementia. Many people worry about this as they get older but it is likely that their memory has never been very good. In dementia we are describing a *change from normal*. Someone who previously had a bad memory for names would get even worse if they had dementia, and all their other mental abilities would fail.

Loss of contact with others caused by deafness, visual impairment, lack of social stimulation or being stuck in bed may make a person so cut off that they appear to be suffering from dementia. We need to be absolutely sure that their condition has been expertly diagnosed, and that these other circumstances have been dealt with.

TREATABLE CONDITIONS IN DEMENTIA

The symptoms associated with dementia are often made worse temporarily by periods of physical ill-health or changes in social circumstance. Not every worsening of confusion or change in behaviour is due to dementia. Indeed, very often these changes are due to causes such as:

- anaemia, diabetes, chest diseases, heart problems, cancer;
- poor nutrition;
- 'cocktails' of drugs (sleeping pills, tranquillisers and anti-depressants);
- discomfort associated with constipation, the pain from bad teeth, bad feet or shingles.

These problems can be treated. Because you work closely with the residents or day care clients, you are in a good position to notice the changes and ask for a doctor to make an expert diagnosis.

BEHAVIOUR

If you did not know the person before their dementia developed, and so do not know very well what their previous personality was like, you may find it difficult to recognise or measure the subtle changes of initiative and vitality and variations in mood that occur, even quite early in dementia. These may be the first and most persistently distressing changes to be appreciated by the family. The person may become 'touchy' or argumentative, banging doors, withdrawing to sulk in bed in a 'blue mood', or lashing out with fists.

Mrs Begum Staff have noticed that Mrs Begum has become irritable. She is clearly troubled about something but refuses to talk about it. The other day she was shouting and accusing staff of stealing her purse, which eventually was found under her pillow. They have also noticed that she seems unable to find her room, although she claims to be just walking. Because she only manages to creep along with a Zimmer frame, these walks are making her very tired.

So-called 'behaviour problems' or 'personality changes' do not by any means happen to everybody with dementia, but when they do happen they cause a lot of distress. The person with dementia may withdraw, to become a 'shadow' or 'shell' of their former self, sitting, staring but apparently seeing nothing, contributing nothing. Or coarseness, lewdness, carelessness and vulgarity may emerge, which are an embarrassment or a hazard or both.

Sometimes people with dementia misinterpret what they see; for example, they imagine that their reflection in the mirror is someone else or that characters on the TV are real and in the room with them. Some experience hallucinations – seeing visions of people, creatures or 'imaginary visitors'. Others become very suspicious of what people are doing behind their backs. Or they may become restless, wandering all the time or repeatedly putting on and taking off their clothes.

Some of this behaviour can be distressing both for relatives, staff and other residents or day care clients and for the person concerned, particularly if they have times when they are lucid and realise that something is happening to them. Other behaviour can seem childlike and be amusing, so there is a temptation to play along with the person. However, we should adopt approaches that show respect for the individual and avoid creating more anxiety and distress.

It is vital that we do not think of all this as part of that person's 'normal self'. These changes can be understood by understanding the changes that are occurring in the control mechanisms of the brain, and by understanding how the individual is reacting to the experience of dementia.

SUPPORT FOR PEOPLE WITH DEMENTIA

It can be difficult to manage alone with such a disabling condition, but people can often continue to live in their own home because someone is there to provide care and protection in this familiar environment. If a husband or wife is still alive and reasonably fit, he or she will almost always provide the necessary care with little complaint and asking for little help unless demands become very great. Mrs Amble, for example, coped for several years with support from her husband. It was only after his death that her dementia became obvious.

Those who are alone because their partner has died or they have never married may move to be with others: daughters, sons, brothers, sisters or friends – and a new 'compensating' household is created.

ADMISSION TO A HOME OR DAY CARE

If there is no safe place within the family household, life 'in care' – in a residential home or nursing home – can become the only option. At least 50 per cent of older people living in Homes are there because dementia has created difficulties for them, like both Mr Ho and Mrs Amble. Nevertheless, we should not think that residential care is a risk-free environment. The person with dementia might be at more risk living with others in strange surroundings than if they stayed in their own home. Why do you think this might be? Think about how you would act if you woke up in a strange bed in a strange room.

As people with dementia are given support and help by the various social and voluntary services to remain in the community longer, you may find that requests for admission to a Home are for vulnerable people with dementia, who seem to be increasingly dependent. The extra challenges and dilemmas they present can tax the range and quality of care that staff can provide.

Day care

People such as Mr Hastie and Miss Peacock do not necessarily need 24-hour residential care but may require respite and day care support. Although both are vulnerable, they are very different individuals and have different living/home circumstances and so require different things from day care. The reasons for their attending day care must be based on diagnosis and on assessment and planned responses.

Diagnosis and assessment

Attendance at day care or admission to a Home is a very important time for people with dementia. They will find change frightening and alarming, and so they need to feel welcomed, safe and secure in a totally strange environment. All too often, other professionals or relatives label the person as having dementia based on flimsy evidence. A doctor's diagnosis therefore is important prior to attendance at day care or admission to residential care.

If you were to meet Mr Ho and Mrs Amble as new residents, it is likely that you would note some similarities in their situation as well as differences. Both have dementia, both are at risk and both may not fully understand where and when or why they are in a nursing home or residential care home.

For the right care to begin at the first meeting, the unique life experience and history of each individual must be recognised. It also requires careful consideration of the particular needs of new residents and day care clients, and not seeing the label of 'dementia' as meaning that a predetermined set of negative responses and attitudes are appropriate. The mainstays of good care are psychological, social and physical therapies, maintained in an environment where the people feel safe and at home, respected and understood.

Despite dementia, people can enjoy life if they are encouraged to exercise, share humour and use long-standing skills. They will feel pleasure and pride, and give both of these to others. Providing the best and most therapeutic lifestyle for each person requires enlightened and dedicated managers and staff.

Assessment

Assessment of the person's needs is crucial and should be done as soon as possible after admission. A thorough assessment should include some reference to general health and any medication they are taking.

Assessment is not all about gathering reams of facts. It is primarily about trying to obtain some understanding of the lifestyle of the person. You can do this by talking with them about what they worked as, or where they lived and who was important for them in their life. This will give you clues to the extent to which they know where they are and will also allow you to have some feeling of involvement in the conversation.

There are a variety of standardised forms that are used to assess factors such as confusion, sociability, understanding and nursing needs. Appendix 2 is a sample of the Extended Crichton Behaviour Rating Scale. Other such scales are the Clifton Assessment Procedures for the Elderly (CAPE) and the Revised Elderly Persons Dependency Scale (REPDS). Most of the forms are completed by asking questions of someone who knows the person best, so they are seldom used on admission. Ideally, the key worker should complete them after the first couple of weeks and then every few months to monitor any improvements or declines.

Assessing levels of ability and competence and how much risk to allow becomes a problem if the individual has some difficulty in communicating with you. For people like Mr Ho and Mrs Amble an assessment of their needs may take longer and may require some creativity on your part to find ways of getting answers to your questions. For people like Mr Hastie and Miss Peacock, who may retain a degree of lucidity, communication may not be such a problem.

Coping with unusual behaviour

Managers usually have to bear in mind the best interests of the existing group when considering a new admission. Some residents or day care clients will tolerate unusual behaviour whereas others will not.

Mrs Amble thinks her bedroom is her council flat, so she walks around the Home dressed for outdoors, handbag and all, continually trying the locked doors to get out.

This is where 'behaviour management' skills come in. Mrs Amble might be persuaded to stay in if there were familiar, domestic activities to keep her occupied or if she were given enough exercise. The solution will depend on a careful analysis of her behaviour and a problem-solving approach. We talk about this more in Chapter 3.

Such behaviour can create problems for you because you can see her frustration, yet there may be no simple solution. If she lacks road sense, but is allowed out of the Home, she could be a risk to herself and others. The solution will depend on your knowledge of Mrs Amble's previous lifestyle and habits and her behaviour in the Home.

An assumption often made by staff is that people with dementia are dependent, requiring to be protected and helped to carry out daily living tasks.

For Mr Hastie and Miss Peacock this clearly may not be the case, so it is important to find out from them why they think they are attending day care.

There will be some people who are very dependent on staff to assist them with daily living tasks, whilst others with encouragement and support may still be able to do simple things for themselves.

To avoid staff becoming like warders with keys, it can often help to give residents and day care clients opportunities to be involved in a purposeful way in doing household chores, or an activity that can distract the individual away from particular repetitive behaviour. But it can be puzzling and frustrating for care staff to hear someone give a very clear account of their past and yet be unable to remember their name or to whom they are speaking. A person can be very able with numbers whilst hopeless with words, unable to get dressed yet brilliant at crosswords.

The care team also face another set of challenges. How do you ensure that your responses to the person with dementia are the right ones, at the right time, in the right way and at the right level of care so as to avoid creating too much dependency? You may feel unduly pressured and lack confidence in dealing with the stressful demands – some of which are unpredictable – of the person with dementia. Your response to such demands may sharply bring into focus the need for some further training.

KEY POINTS

- As people age, they are generally slower of thought and emotion – this does not necessarily mean that they have dementia.

- Difficulty with memory, particularly for recent events, is the hallmark of dementia.

- Memory problems are not the only changes that occur; loss of emotional control, strange beliefs and experiences, aggression or fear may be more apparent at some times.

- Dementia is most common in very old people and is probably the main reason that very old people move into care. Nevertheless, many people with dementia continue to live in their own homes until they have serious difficulties in coping on their own.

- Medicines, chest complaints and other physical illnesses can create dementia-like symptoms. These are treatable but require a medical assessment by a doctor.

- The two most common dementias – Alzheimer's disease and multi-infarct dementia – have different characteristics, but both are progressive and often bring forward death.

- Managers and staff have a crucial role in setting standards of care.

- A rigorous assessment and review process is needed to monitor changes in the person with dementia.

- For people with dementia, living in a group setting may prompt further disturbing behaviour.

TRAINING EXERCISE

On admission, Mr Ho gives you concern because of his lethargy and his apparent inability to communicate in English. He has reverted to his first learnt language and has stopped communicating in English. This poses serious problems for staff if they do not know Cantonese, as well as for Mr Ho because he seems to think that he is living in Hong Kong as a young man.

What course of action might you take?

2 Understanding and Care

In some ways, people who suffer from dementia are just like other people. They are adults with the same rights as other adults – the right to their own privacy, the right to make decisions for themselves, the right to respect from others. In some ways, though, they differ. In this chapter we look at those differences, because understanding will help us to care for people with dementia in a way that allows for their difficulties.

SAME ILLNESS, DIFFERENT SYMPTOMS

In Chapter 1 we noted that differences are sometimes due to the ways in which different causes of dementia affect the brain. In vascular dementia, strokes are common and the person may need special help with mobility (getting about) or with speech problems. In dementia associated with Parkinson's disease (Lewy body dementia), mobility problems are again common but there are also hallucinations, which may present particular problems. Even within one type of dementia such as Alzheimer's disease, different people are affected differently because different bits of the brain seem to be more or less affected. Some people have had memory problems and only memory problems for years. Other difficulties have only come late on in the illness. Some people have great difficulties in coping with skills such as dressing from quite early on in the illness, yet for others it is the change of personality that is most obvious. Of course, active people with mild dementia present their carers with problems different from those posed by people in the final stages who need almost constant nursing care.

ALLOWING FOR DIFFICULTIES

'I' as a person am a combination of understanding, memory, actions, emotions and conscience, which decline in dementia. People who develop dementia become less than themselves, and can behave like children or in other ways we do not expect. There are a few similarities between people with dementia and children; indeed, they may eventually become as dependent physically as the youngest infant. There are even people with dementia who quite like being treated in a childish way (there are, after all, people like that who do not have dementia!). But they are *not* children, and most of them would like us to treat them as they actually are – older adults with a wealth of past experience who are very slowly dying from a tragic illness.

So people with dementia are not children who are making mistakes and need to be corrected so that they learn. They are adults with whole lifetimes of experience behind them – indeed, usually much more experience of life than we, their carers, have. How do we remember to treat someone with dignity if that person cannot remember all their past life or has lost their own sense of self-respect? The answer is that we constantly remind ourselves of who they were before this illness struck. Think about:

- how the person would like to have been treated if they had not lost their memory;
- the person's present abilities;
- the person's social graces.

If the person cannot tell us much about their past life, their family and friends will fill in some, if not all, of the gaps. They will also tell of those little islands of normality that often happen in dementia, when suddenly an old memory is recovered, a name from the past is mentioned or the person acts as if they were still at work. It also may help if we try to put ourselves in the individual's position: how would we like to be treated if we were having these difficulties?

CHANGES

The changes that occur in dementia do not happen all at once. They are very gradual and differences may not be noticed over just a month or two. Staff in care homes and day centres will only occasionally see people at the very beginning of the process, very slowly beginning to lose their memory.

What happens next varies from person to person. In some people, memory loss is the most obvious change. In others, it is a decline in their ability to care for themselves. In others still, it is their ability to communicate or their social graces that decline most obviously. Some people continue to be able to carry out quite complicated actions, or to remember a few very fixed old memories, or to keep their personality till quite late, when all their other abilities are long since gone. Why these differences happen is not entirely clear – it may be that different parts of the brain are damaged more at an early stage in some people than others. Whatever individual differences there are, however, the overall process of dementia is the same slow decline till the person dies.

UNDERSTANDING BRAIN FUNCTIONING

The human brain can be likened to a complex control centre or a computer that has many different parts and functions but essentially is programmed to enable us to cope and deal with the demands of daily living. So our brain is the means by which we:

- have understanding;
- have memory;
- control our actions;
- express emotions;
- have a conscience.

The brain, as the control centre for the human body, receives all the signals, stimuli and information that we gain from what we see, hear, smell, touch and taste. Our senses play an important part in gaining this information, and the brain processes it so that we can understand what is happening round about us. Of course, we are constantly receiving lots of different signals at the same time, so the brain acts as a filter to help us focus on what is important for us at that moment.

The illness of dementia does not cause loss of eyesight or hearing, though older people may have poor eyesight or hearing for completely different reasons. What goes wrong is the way in which the brain makes sense of all the information it receives.

This means that some people with dementia will see and hear perfectly well but:

- may be unable to make sense of what they see;
- may be disorientated in the Home or day centre and have no sense of time;
- may not understand what is happening;
- may be unable to make sense of what is being spoken to them or what they hear;
- may have difficulty in recognising close relatives.

Loss of awareness

Mr Ho became very agitated, restless and abruptly pushed away staff who went to help him. He neither ate nor slept for a couple of days, and his key worker reported her concerns to the manager of the Home.

Sometimes people with dementia may know there is something wrong with them and, because they cannot understand the sensations coming from their own body, they become agitated. It is likely that Mr Ho felt ill and was in pain but, because of his dementia, he did not make sense of what was happening to him and so could not tell anyone. It was therefore crucial that his key worker knew she had to interpret Mr Ho's behaviour and try to make sense of why he was distressed, agitated and not eating or sleeping. She suggested to the manager that the doctor should be called in, as she felt it might be a physical problem. The GP discovered that Mr Ho had a urinary tract infection, and with medication he returned to his old self.

Gradually you have to begin to fill in the gaps in the individual's understanding, but not to the extent of taking over all decisions and tasks of daily living. Each person should be encouraged to use their remaining faculties as much as possible, and your help should be given only when they are ready to be helped.

Memory

Another main function of the brain is to store information in such a way that it can be used again. This can be likened to a bank in which we deposit our money or savings. We withdraw from our savings account when we need the resources (money) to purchase something. Our memory can be thought of as a resources bank: when we find ourselves in a strange, new or unfamiliar situation, we draw on previous experience to enable us to cope.

The different *types* of memory we have are for:

- words;
- events;
- people's faces;
- personal life history;
- actions;
- things learnt at school;
- things learnt at work;
- all social skills;
- music;
- pictures.

This enormous store of past knowledge, skills and experience is called on for everything to do with day-to-day living.

But we also have different *time-scales* of memory. We do not remember everything for ever! To dial a telephone number requires a few seconds of memory which in most cases can then be forgotten. But to recall where the car is parked, or the reason for coming shopping or where the house keys were left, demands a longer-lasting sort of memory.

From the earliest stages of the disease, a person with dementia will have difficulty, especially with recent memories. Later, all memories are gradually lost: they disappear from the store, or, if they are still in the store, they cannot be retrieved.

You will gradually become the person's 'memory'. Reminders such as a diary or a scrapbook of memories, a photograph or a special ornament or article can be used to prompt important memories. The resident or day care client will want to use their own reminders in their own way and in their own time as well as those created by staff. In Chapter 3 we talk about this in more detail.

Connections

The third function of the brain is also its most complicated. A lot of the huge volume of the brain is there to make incredibly complicated connections between different bits of information coming from outside or stored in the memory. Functions such as thinking, dreaming, imagining, solving problems and understanding all gradually decline in dementia. For the individual with dementia it might begin with just a little difficulty in solving new complicated problems. This will eventually progress to a complete loss of the person's mental abilities.

You may have to make up for these losses by simplifying the decisions that the person has to make, and later gradually taking over decision-making when it becomes necessary. If possible the individual should be involved in handing over to others control of making decisions, and should be encouraged to retain their independence to the last possible moment. Insist on taking over only if there are major risks apparent. There is not much wrong in people with dementia taking mistaken decisions if no one, especially they themselves, gets hurt. Mr Hastie, for example, likes to take his tea from a thermos flask and his sandwiches from a lunchbox. He often takes his tea at the wrong time but staff simply replenish the flask so he is not alarmed when he gives himself another tea-break.

Actions

The brain directs actions. Everything in day-to-day living – such as washing, dressing, eating, going to the toilet, housework, shopping, work, social activities and interests, speaking and writing, emotional and sexual behaviour, even moving muscles to walk, sit or stand – is controlled by some part of the brain. All these actions will gradually decline. This may begin with difficulties in complicated actions such as driving or operating machinery at work, or with little mistakes in dressing. Later, all the individual's abilities decline. But remember that by prompting the individual you can help them to retain their limited ability.

Gradually, you will need more and more to fill in the gaps in the person's physical abilities. In the last stages of dementia an individual will be completely dependent on the care given by people around them.

Emotions

The brain is involved in emotional feelings, including the ability to be interested in things or motivated to do things. Gradually the person with dementia seems to feel less strongly about things, and becomes less interested in getting involved in old or new activities. This can be very frustrating for carers, but is an inevitable part of the illness. You need to learn not to expect too much emotional response.

Frontal lobe functioning

The front part of the brain is called the frontal lobe. It has the very important function of acting as a 'moderator' of our actions. Whether we carry out actions in the course of our daily living is based on learnt norms or what is considered acceptable by ourselves and others. All of us as individuals have a standard against which we:

- plan and think ahead;
- monitor our actions to check whether we are doing things correctly;
- check something we have completed to see whether we did it right or wrong.

Even the simple task of turning on a gas cooker involves each step being compared with a standard. We learn that, to light the gas, we need to plan to have matches and that we do not turn the gas tap on until we have the matches! We check that, once the match is struck, the gas actually lights. These comparisons with a standard are made in everything we do, from simple tasks to moral decisions about what is right or wrong.

Mrs Begum has tried to befriend Mrs Amble because she has become concerned that Mrs Amble seems unable to take care of her personal hygiene. Staff also have noticed that Mrs Amble is not keeping herself clean, is not washing herself, is refusing to brush her hair and is wearing the same clothes every day. Mrs Begum became quite upset when, on one occasion, Mrs Amble decided to strip off in the sitting room in full view of the male residents.

Dementia causes some individuals like Mrs Amble to lose their standards in personal appearance, sense of right and wrong or their control over their actions. However, we must treat the individual concerned with respect and sensitivity, and not adopt an over-strict, overbearing manner about the incident. Remember that Mrs Amble may not understand that she is doing anything out of the ordinary. On the other hand, people should not be left to do very embarrassing things or things that hurt or offend other residents or day care clients. As a staff member you may have to intervene but not to the extent of stopping someone in your care being in control of their life and actions.

A good response to Mrs Amble's actions would have been for the staff member to explain that the sitting room was not her bedroom, and to ask if she wanted to get undressed for a reason and then take her to the bedroom. It might also be important to explain to Mrs Begum why Mrs Amble behaved in this way.

FEELINGS MATTER!

Another very important aspect of dementia is how the people with the disease see themselves and their illness as it progresses towards death. It might be expected that it would be terrifying and depressing; yet some people seem to be blissfully unaware of their dementia. You may be tempted to assume that no one who suffers from dementia knows their situation and so you need not bother with their feelings. Nothing could be further from the truth.

In the early stages of dementia, and for some people even at more advanced stages, their experience of dementia can mean feeling depressed or worried or frustrated or embarrassed or just bewildered.

Being unsure of the place that staff say is 'home' or who these strangers called 'staff' are can be extremely frustrating and bewildering. If there is no recollection of when a move happened, or the reason for it, a resident may well feel very distressed. Mrs Amble is clearly distressed by her failing memory although she tries to conceal it.

Mrs Amble's key worker, Mary, is worried. Mrs Amble is beginning to behave in odd ways. She keeps asking who the strangers in her home are – 'these funny old people who want to sleep in my house' – and she has taken to locking herself into her bedroom and hoarding her possessions. The other day when Mary was helping Mrs Amble brush her hair, Mary had brought a mirror for her to look into and commented 'You're all ready for a night on the town – and you look so young with your new hairdo no one would know you are 85.' Mrs Amble became very angry and shouted at Mary that she was not 85, that the woman's face in the mirror was her mother – she was 35, and tearfully asked when she was going home from this nice hotel.

Many people like Mrs Amble who have dementia are so bewildered by the whole experience that they seem not to react at all; they retreat into themselves, and act as if nothing unusual was happening.

It is important to try to recognise how she is actually feeling, to react sensitively to these feelings and not to dismiss them as just part of the illness. For Mrs Amble, having dementia and being upset by what she is experiencing are quite likely to cause her to do things that we find hard to understand. She may:

- hoard her possessions because she is afraid of losing them or that they will be stolen;
- withdraw into herself and her past memories and not take part in things because she is too embarrassed and does not understand;
- keep trying to find her own home in order to look for people who understand and care;
- get angry at staff (who are, to her, strangers) attempting to help her;
- not recognise herself in a mirror or recent photograph because she cannot remember getting older.

Recognising the many different feelings that people with dementia may experience can help us understand their behaviour and so respond in more helpful ways.

Miss Peacock upsets residents in the lounge because of her interfering behaviour. She disturbs them by continually rearranging newspapers, ornaments and their personal belongings. The residents complain that she is bossy and does not allow them to do what they want. The care staff are talked down to and called 'nurses', and she does not seem to be prepared to listen to what they say.

The activities organiser reminded care staff that Miss Peacock had been a carer herself, and suggested that perhaps she could be encouraged to help with some of the daily chores. In fact, care staff recognised that, despite her confusion, one or two residents seemed to be stimulated by her gossip and bossy attitude. It was decided that the activities worker would arrange for Miss Peacock to help with organising and planning the day care activities. Within a few days, Miss Peacock seemed to be more contented and was less disruptive of the activities of the other residents.

DEMENTIA AFFECTS THE FAMILY TOO

Dementia is an illness that is just as devastating, or more so, for those who love the person most. Relatives or spouses often have to watch the person change gradually from what they were, becoming more and more helpless, losing their energy and personality, and gradually losing touch with the reality around them. They will notice those odd changes in personality, or the strange behaviour.

For the close relative or friend of someone with dementia, this will be like a bereavement. The person with dementia is mentally dying before them, although their body stays healthy till quite late on in the illness. It will be depressing and distressing. It is made worse by the fact that many people with dementia lose the ability to respond to their family's distress. In addition, families have often been stuck in this caring position for a long time before the person has to come into care, perhaps unwillingly. The Ho family soldiered on for a long time coping with Mr Ho's decline and their own distress before he came into the Home.

The Ho family are similar to most families caring for someone with dementia. They found the experience extremely stressful and it aroused many different emotions. Not only did they not understand what was happening to Mr Ho; they also had mixed reactions and feelings about his behaviour and the idea of his moving into care. They felt guilty that they could not keep on caring, distressed by Mr Ho's reactions, but relieved and grateful for the care being offered.

Families and friends need to know as much as they can about dementia, its causes and symptoms. They may want to continue to be involved in the care of their relative or friend and this should be possible. They should have access to support from staff, perhaps in the form of a regular support group. Mr Ho's family, for example, are realising that he is increasingly living in the past. He makes sense of the Home in terms of his early adulthood in Hong Kong. His family have therefore agreed to provide the sort of food he would have eaten. One of them comes in once a day and cooks and eats a conventional Chinese meal with him. This has helped the mentally alert residents, the staff and the relatives' group to understand the implications of memory loss in dementia.

THE EXPERIENCE OF THE INDIVIDUAL

For some people, attending day care or coming into a Home is likely to be an admission of defeat. For Mr Hastie and Miss Peacock, they might realise for the first time that they are 'failing'. This is particularly so if they thought they were being completely independent at home, if they did not see what their relatives saw – that they were not looking after themselves, that they were being dangerous with the cooker, or wandering out and getting lost, or that they were just sitting doing nothing all day and were miserable. Some individuals will be able to come to terms with the 'defeat' of day care or admission to a Home, but many will not. They never saw themselves as the sort of people who gave up; they never thought they would need to go into a Home or to accept 'charity', and they may have been under considerable pressure from family, doctors, social workers to attend day care or stay in a Home. Mrs Amble illustrates this, and her behaviour on admission showed how upset she was although she was unable to say so.

They may forget that they agreed to come in, or feel that they did not consent. When they do come in, the experience will be far more puzzling for a person with dementia than for other individuals. They may expect to be going home again, or think this is their home, or think they are in somewhere other than a care home, such as a hotel (like Mrs Amble).

HELPING ORIENTATION

This needs your time and patience. Everything has to be repeated many times, for people with dementia can, with prompting, learn things slowly. Visual clues, such as clearly marked toilet doors or pictures to signify the dining room or bedroom, can help the new resident find their way around the Home. You might like to give the person with dementia a downstairs bedroom that is easy to see.

Nevertheless, some will never learn their way around, and a decision has to be taken to guide them when they need to move from one place to another. No one should be left lost in the middle of a strange place without help just because we believe that they should be as independent as possible.

KEY POINTS

- People with dementia are adults with a whole lifetime of experience behind them.
- Every person with dementia has an individual pathway through the illness.
- Care staff should be sensitive to the differing needs of individuals.
- People with dementia should be encouraged to retain a degree of independence, however limited that might be.
- People with dementia may not understand that certain actions or types of behaviour are inappropriate or upsetting for others.

■ Families and friends should be encouraged to maintain relationships and be involved in some of the caring tasks.

TRAINING EXERCISE

What is the experience of someone with dementia in your centre or Home? Think of someone coming into care for the first time. Perhaps they had accepted some help in their own home – home carers, Meals on Wheels, sitter services? If they did, then they had already made the first step in accepting that they cannot do everything for themselves.

What can you do to help that person retain some sense of personal worth and value?

3 Working with Dementia

This chapter looks at ways that you can provide therapeutic care for someone with dementia. It discusses many of the difficulties, such as the attitudes of residents or day care clients who do *not* have dementia and the fact that some people refuse to be helped. The key to positive care is knowing the person well, and life story books are suggested as a good way of achieving this.

All types of dementia are due to deterioration in the brain. Many of its symptoms, such as memory loss and loss of the ability to care for oneself, are common to all sufferers. But all sufferers are individual people, and are very different from each other.

DIFFERENT PEOPLE, DIFFERENT REACTIONS

As well as the differences due to the varying effects of the illness, the people who suffer from dementia had different 'starting points'. They come from different educational and social backgrounds, different races and religions, and they bring different personality characteristics with them. These personality characteristics matter a great deal in our understanding of how to work with a person with dementia.

- Some people who have always been very active mentally will want to know what is going on, will require things to occupy their mind and may resent the inactivity that dementia can bring – for example, being unable to read or to knit.

- Others who are naturally more easy-going may be prepared to sit around not doing a great deal.
- Some people who have prided themselves on their independence may resent having to rely on care staff for help.
- Others may be passive and enjoy being looked after.
- Some people who have always had high standards may dislike not being able to remember where their clothes or the knives and forks belong.
- Others who are more untidy by nature do not notice the change in themselves so much.
- Some people enjoy a lot of company.
- Others prefer their own company.

Most people with dementia will continue to be the people they were, though a few will suffer a personality change. It is only in the later stages of the illness that significant personality changes occur.

WHO WERE THEY?

We need to know a lot about the sorts of people they have been all their lives before we can begin to work with individuals who have dementia. This knowledge will explain a lot of the differences between people; it will help us to understand how someone reacts to the illness and to attending a day centre or living in care with others. It will give us ideas about their attitudes, interests, likes and dislikes. We will learn whom they are likely to get on with, something about how they might want to spend their time and what their reactions to difficulties will be. Mr Hastie, for example, is used to being busy, being outside and being with men. Activities specifically for men are not always provided in day care. Carole Archibald's book *Activities 2* includes suggested activities for men.

Life story books

As well as knowing what type of person an individual has been, we need to know details about how they have spent their previous life. When we first meet someone with dementia, we know little of their background, even if there has been a proper assessment or a social or medical background report. The person may not be able now to remember all the details of their past life, and relatives may not be available to fill in the details.

One of the first tasks should be to fill in these gaps. One method is to create a 'life story book', a scrapbook that will actually contain all that is known about this person. It will usually have information on where they were born and brought up, who their family were, where they were taught and what their school was like, what jobs they did and who they worked with, what their hobbies and interests were, and what their social life was like. There will also be details of important relationships, marriage, children, grandchildren, etc, and a lot about where they have lived. It will almost always contain important information about their interests, beliefs and attitudes. It should have copies of any photographs, letters or other documents that throw light on that person's life, work and relationships. It is in fact like an imaginative 'This is Your Life' feature.

Not all life story books will have such a lot of information. A few people do not wish to recall their personal lives and prefer their life story books to focus on an important part of their lives such as their football club, their old regiment or their days in the Women's Land Army. Miss Peacock will want pictures of the hospital in which she worked as well as pictures of her mother.

It is very important that, as far as possible, the person with dementia takes part in the exercise, writing in what they remember, visiting old haunts with a member of staff who takes a camera to record the visit, asking relatives for items of information or material for the book. And it is vital that the book is not just made up and then left. It is there most for the individual to use, guided by staff; it is there to add new information to; it is there to help the family to reminisce with their relative; and it is there to remind the staff constantly that this is not just a person with dementia, this is a person with a past history and past experiences which have been important to them and which have made them the person they are.

Mr Ho's key worker and his family prepared a life story book. They used a photograph album with clear plastic to cover the photographs because many of them were very precious to the family. They showed Mr Ho's life before he came to Britain and his subsequent take-away and restaurant businesses. Special terms and Chinese quotations were included. There were no photographs of his present family because the family explained that, by Chinese tradition, photographs are used only when people are dead. Captions were in Chinese and English so that Mr Ho's key worker could sit with him and talk about the contents, as could his family.

Life story books can provide a thoroughly enjoyable one-to-one activity. Leafing through the pages and sharing memories gives relatives something they can do again and again because the person with dementia cannot usually remember the last time. You can use the books to soothe an anxious or agitated person or perhaps to distract them from more troublesome activity. A session of intimate sharing can improve confidence and self-esteem – yours as well as theirs.

PERSONAL SPACE

People with dementia are very individual and you can emphasise that individuality in the way you treat them. But there are some ways in which the person with dementia can be in danger of being set apart from other residents or day care clients who do not suffer from dementia.

The way this happens will depend partly on whether the residents or day care clients know and like the person with dementia. Mrs Begum, for example, is a well liked resident. She went through an unhappy period when she realised her memory was going, but settled again afterwards. She is increasingly confused but very friendly so is not a problem to other residents. Mrs Amble, on the other hand, is shunned because she is neither known nor liked. These two residents illustrate how important the group as a whole is in many respects, including the influence it may have on the way staff deal with people with dementia.

Mrs Begum has begun to feel that the restless and agitated behaviour of Mrs Amble is disturbing her quiet times. Matters came to a head when Mrs Begum discovered Mrs Amble in her bedroom, rummaging through her personal possessions and throwing things on to the floor. Mrs Begum was quite shocked and told Mrs Amble that she should leave her room, but Mrs Amble became angry, abusive, and shouted at Mrs Begum that this was her room and refused to leave.

Such situations are likely to occur in Homes or day care centres where there are individuals with dementia and more mentally alert people. Some of the 'normal' people may feel that those with dementia get too much staff attention. They may feel impatient with the person who continually repeats a question or some action, or mistakes them for a long-lost relative; or, like Mrs Begum, may become frightened when they intrude into their bedroom. If not dealt with properly, the people with dementia will find that they are overly criticised, shunned by others and regarded as a nuisance. This can become much worse if staff also have similar prejudices and reactions.

To some extent the answer to this problem is to try to prevent it. In general it is probably better for care homes either to specialise in dementia care only or to have separate specialist units for people with dementia. Alternatively, if it is a general needs Home, there could be an admissions policy that keeps the number of people with dementia below about 30 per cent of the total. Homes need to have very clear policies about how they will deal with the individual who is very disturbed in their behaviour. However, it is not always possible to avoid difficult mixes of people.

BRIDGING GAPS

Attempts should be made to bridge the gap between people with dementia and those without. Mentally alert people need to learn about dementia and its consequences, as they may not have realised that they would be mixing with people with dementia when they agreed to come into your Home or day centre. They need to know that it is not catching and to have a chance to talk about their feelings of fear, anxiety, anger and frustration. Involve them if possible in looking at the life story books. This can help them see that these people, who may now seem rude or aggressive or interfering, were originally people just like them but have now been changed by their illness. They should be encouraged to take part in helping the individuals with dementia to understand where they are and to be involved in activities where possible.

By ensuring that the individuals with dementia are treated as adults and given respect and affection, whilst involving the mentally alert people in shared activities, fears can be diminished on both sides and the gap can be bridged.

In many cases it will be difficult for the two groups of residents or day care clients to communicate and feel at home with each other all the time. A break from each other can be helpful for both groups.

Mrs Begum Mrs Ali, the care worker for Mrs Begum, had noticed her increased frustration and agitation because of the disturbance caused by Mrs Amble's behaviour in the Home. Mrs Ali thought that a break from the resident group might be helpful. So she arranged that she would go with Mrs Begum to visit her family, who would then take her to the local temple. This special activity helped Mrs Begum to recognise that she was as important as Mrs Amble.

NO ONE SINGLE APPROACH!

There are great differences between one person and another in how the illness of dementia affects their lifestyle, personality and behaviour. What has already been said about the great differences between one person and another in their dementia should immediately make us realise that there is no one single approach to caring for people with dementia. There are, however, a few important and useful ideas.

Creating a sense of belonging

The most important principle of all is that, for many activities, there really is no reason to think of people with dementia as any different from anybody else. When there is a dance or a sing-song, when we are talking about the news or the past or the weather, or visiting a museum or a park, or going on a holiday, or when we are asking residents or day care clients about their views about the service we are providing – indeed in all the activities that a good care home or day centre will regularly be engaged in – there is no reason why many people with dementia should be excluded, and no reason why they should not be able to play a part. Some minor allowances may have to be made: for difficulties in keeping up with what is going on, for repetitiveness, for poor coordination. But most people with dementia will appreciate the feeling that they are not being put to one side, and that the rest of the residents or day care clients and staff treat them as ordinary people.

We can, though, carry our wish for normality too far. If a person with dementia is confused by an activity, or gets distressed, or is so disturbed that they disrupt proceedings, it is not much help to anybody. It increases the feelings of distrust among those who do not have dementia, and it damages the morale of the individual with dementia.

Focus on retained abilities

It is all too easy to think immediately of the disabilities that the person with dementia experiences rather than of the abilities they still have. It is likely that your assessment of needs will focus on the negative ways of looking at individuals. This 'deficit model' approach does very little to help us feel optimistic about an individual's future and is demoralising for staff. Consequently, it makes us take over too soon and often we treat the person like a dependent child.

People with dementia usually retain some of a particular ability, as all brain functioning is not affected until late in the illness. This means that some of your residents or day care clients may still be able to knit, do the crossword, play snooker, discuss politics, play cards, bet on horses quite successfully, recite poetry, play a musical instrument. Yet they may not be able to dress or wash themselves without some assistance.

Do not assume that, because they can do one skilful task, they will be able to look after themselves totally if they are given time or space. Some individuals will require a minimum of prompting and get there in time whilst others will really need help and support.

Adequate stimulation

Many people with dementia lose their motivation and energy, and tend to sit about for long periods. This can often be a result of their awareness that they:

- are likely to say the wrong thing;
- forget where they are;
- forget who they are talking to.

It has also shown that just teaching what time of day it is is not much help. If we are to be successful in helping people to orientate themselves better, the individuals themselves need to be involved, by using their senses to help see what kind of day it is, by actively practising how to find the toilet, or by helping fill up the diary.

Although reality orientation does not have much to offer people who have more severe dementia, it is most helpful with those who have only mild dementia and are 'nearly orientated'. Most of all, it has made us all realise that how we as staff or relatives approach and talk to people with dementia actually matters.

Reminiscing

Many (though not all) older people enjoy taking time to reminisce, to review their past life, reliving the high spots, putting it all in perspective, giving thanks for past good times. Some dwell a bit too much on past failures and family squabbles. A few use their recollection of the past to show how unhappy they are now. Most people can get a sense of fulfilment and well-being through their reminiscence, even if it occasionally involves a little self-deception.

For the person with dementia who has lost touch with most of the present and who may feel they are not very competent in the present, looking back can bring back that sense of reality and that sense of competence. It can be a real morale-booster. Not only that. Sometimes we find that reminiscence actually reminds the person of something that they are still able to do but had forgotten about.

Life story books are the key to good reminiscence work but other activities can be helpful, too. Playing old music, singing old songs, reading old newspapers and books, and going to old haunts, museum collections, oral history projects, 'reminiscence theatre' where actors play out the memories that individuals tell them about, can all be stimulating and bring the person back to life. They also reinforce that important message to staff – this is not 'another grey-haired demented old lady with glasses', it is a real person with a long and interesting past history.

Just as with all the ideas in this chapter, we must be careful with reminiscence. Not everybody has had a happy life; some have memories they would rather forget. Some find the past distressing and confusing. Reminiscence is not for them.

Validation

'Validation' is basically a way of seeing everything that a person with dementia says or does as being meaningful – it is valid even if it is not obvious to us.

The idea of validation rose out of attempts to understand the odd things that people with dementia say and the odd things that they do. For example, if a resident asks for her mother, is it not likely that she is feeling insecure in the Home? Perhaps she has had a particular fear of being 'put away' or had been in a Home as a child. Maybe she is frightened by the people around her. If you can translate the odd words into an understandable feeling, you can help her insecurity, or you can talk round her feelings about care, or you can try to help her get more used to her fellow residents.

If she is wandering off 'to work', is she feeling bored with the inactivity of her day, or is she feeling that she is not being treated with the respect she used to get at work, or is she feeling guilty at not doing something useful? Again, this translation of odd behaviour into common-sense understanding of her feelings can help us help her to be more settled. Does she need more to do? Do you need to alter your approach to her so that she feels more valued? Do you need to reassure her that she is not doing anything wrong and that it is all right for her to 'put her feet up' and be retired, or be looked after?

Miss Peacock is always complaining about ineffective staff. It might be worth getting her to talk more about this one day and responding to the feeling as well as the words. The chances are that Miss Peacock feels utterly helpless. She failed to prevent her mother leaving and she now has none of the power and authority she had when she was working.

Like reality orientation and reminiscence, validation may not be suitable for everybody. But the ideas behind it are good and should help us to treat residents and day care clients with more respect. In particular, it should help us to understand and help disturbed people more positively than we have in the past.

Listening and responding

When people are anxious, sad or worried it is natural to want to talk over these concerns with a friend, a relative or an outside adviser. However, it is often assumed that people with dementia cannot be helped in this way. So instead of listening, relatives and staff answer the person's anxieties with a sort of general 'It will be all right, dear', which is meaningless, patronising and quickly forgotten.

It is of course true that some people with dementia do quickly forget the reassurance they are given, and may also forget their worries quickly. Others may not be fully able to express what their worries are about but may have strong feelings that affect how they behave. Some may seem to have unrealistic worries but, by using validation, we can try to understand what is worrying them. But it is not true that all people with dementia are unable to discuss their fears and worries, and be helped by doing so.

For example, many people in the early stages of dementia want help to understand what is happening to them, want to know the diagnosis and its consequences, want advice and help about planning their future. Many people with dementia need to talk over at length their loss of independence and loss of control over their lives – as happens when they first need a home care assistant, or first have to ask for help with bills, or first need help with dressing, or have to give up their home to move into care.

The death of a life partner can worsen the person's feeling and sense of loss. These problems are made much worse if a person forgets that they have lost their relative, or their home. Each time you talk to them you may be making them face the loss afresh. But with patience and persistence, people in the early and even middle stages of dementia can learn that they have experienced these losses and also come to terms with the losses to some extent. You certainly should try to help, if the alternative is that the person is in constant distress wondering where their house or their spouse is, or wondering why people are doing things for them that they think they can do themselves.

Helping with distress starts with listening, and by allowing the person to express their distress, not brushing them off with meaningless phrases such as 'there, there, it's all right'. It continues with trying to understand the distress, and then helping the person see how they can work through it and recover, particularly by reorganising their life and filling the gap left by the person, or the ability, they have lost. Unfortunately, some people with dementia seem to get stuck for long periods in a distressed state, and nothing you can do seems to help. But this is only a small minority – most can be understood, advised and reassured.

Diversion

If your attempts to get the person involved in useful, stimulating activity, or your efforts at orientation, or your support and counselling are getting nowhere, you should remember that people with dementia have a poor concentration span, and may forget distress quite soon. Sometimes it is best to change the subject, to divert the person's attention onto some other activity or conversation away from what is distressing them. This can be a very useful technique as long as it is not used in every circumstance, but is seen as a last resort if your attempts to ease a distressing situation are increasing, rather than reducing, the distress.

Mr Hastie Care staff have found that Mr Hastie has periods of distress, agitation and anger. He walks round the Home, slamming doors and hitting the walls with his hands, and he has been found trying to lift the linoleum in the dining room. When staff try to approach him, he raises his fists at them. Despite trying to coax him to have a cup of tea, to distract him, matters do not improve.

As things did not improve with Mr Hastie, the Home's manager and care staff met to review his care plan and to decide what other responses could be tried. During the discussion it emerged that his disruptive behaviour always happened at the same time every day. It was therefore decided that, as he enjoyed going for walks, the outreach worker would ensure that he was always out of the Home at the 'problem' time.

Behaviour therapy

Clinical psychologists have been trying to see if they can develop quite specific ways to help people with dementia who have more extreme behaviour problems, such as repeated aggression, continuous wandering, repetitive shouting, uncontrollable distress. To some extent the psychologists find that using the principles we have discussed above brings good results in most cases. But there are instances where more formal 'behaviour therapy' can help.

This approach starts from a specific, detailed recording of the particular behaviour problem. The recording should detail clearly when, where, how often and under what circumstances it happens. Such an approach can help you gain a whole picture of what is happening for the particular individual. If a psychologist is to be involved in devising some strategies, you have an important part to play in presenting this information. It can give the psychologist some idea of how a change in those circumstances, or in our response to the person's behaviour, could help. These are specialised techniques and need a lot of effort and cooperation by staff because they work only when all staff are involved and treat the person in exactly the same way. It is a good idea to ask the advice of a clinical psychologist if an individual has more severe behaviour problems. As a rough general rule, it is likely that the psychologist will be more able to help if it is one particular type of behaviour that is the problem, rather than general disorganisation of behaviour.

Drugs

Drug therapy is bottom of the list of ideas on how to help a person with dementia. Unfortunately, it is often seen as the first choice, but there is no excuse for the old idea some doctors seemed to have that everybody with dementia should be given a tranquilliser. Nowadays the emphasis is on specific treatments for specific problems. A good doctor will ask you to ensure that all other avenues of therapy have been tried. Staff should always ask themselves if they could learn to be more tolerant of a resident's behaviour. Often you will find that most of the staff can, but one or two find it more difficult. They then need the support of the other staff (not criticism) to help cope better. Often a problem, even an apparently severe one, is only temporary – a few sleepless nights, a brief restless period.

Drugs should be used only when a problem is established over a period – we all have off days and off weeks. Most important of all, any drug treatment that is started must be reviewed regularly, under medical supervision, and stopped as soon as possible, with trial stopping periods to test if it is still necessary.

Drugs may be necessary if a person's sleep pattern has become so disrupted by their dementia that their body does not seem to know when to be asleep and when awake. Drugs may be necessary when it has been proved that physical illness is not the cause of distress or disturbance, and when other attempts to relieve it have failed. An anti-depressant can relieve the depression that is common in early cases, and an anti-anxiety drug in cases where severe anxiety is making the person more confused than they need to be. Some anti-depressants seem to help people who are forced by their dementia to repeat actions endlessly, or who lose control of their emotions, and anti-psychotic drugs may help some who have hallucinations or severely mistaken ideas or delusions. Drugs may even have a place in helping people to settle into a new strange environment which they find confusing and distressing. It is wrong to say that drugs have no place in the treatment of dementia but right to say that they have been over-used in the past. Drugs are not a substitute for proper understanding, care and attention.

COMPLEX INDIVIDUALS

Dealing with people with dementia is a complex but interesting job. Many of them will take part fully in the general programme of activities in a day centre or Home, but many will have to be assessed so that you can provide for their more individual needs.

In devising care plans which cope with that person's problems and take account of their remaining abilities, we should remember the useful part that relatives and friends can play and include them in our plans. We should never be shy of asking for outside help – from general practitioner or community nursing staff, social services staff, occupational therapists and physiotherapists, clinical psychologists, community psychiatric nurses and hospital specialists. There is also a vast range of community resources – libraries, museums, theatres, parks, schools, etc – to which every citizen, including those with dementia, and including those who happen to live in care homes, have right of access.

'Refusers'

One group of people have not been mentioned. With the best programme in the world, with the best staff, with all the encouragement from relatives, with all the expert advice we can get, we have to admit that some people with dementia simply do not want our care plans or our ideas of what would help. They may not understand why, their pride may prevent their joining in, snobbery sometimes gets in the way, they may be too sensitive about their lost abilities or their poor communication, or they may find that they cannot concentrate well enough. Whatever the reason, we must respect this and make arrangements for the refusers whenever we set up any activity, outing or recreation.

KEY POINTS

- Different individuals have different reactions to dementia.
- In mixed resident groups, mentally alert residents should be helped to understand about dementia.
- 'Therapies' work only if the individual is involved actively.
- Significant people and agencies with whom the individual has had contact can support the day care or residential care task.

TRAINING EXERCISE

A number of suggestions were made in Chapter 3 about how staff might respond to individuals. As an exercise, think of someone with dementia whom you are caring for and ask yourself the following questions:

1 Do I really know about this person's previous lifestyle? If not, how can I begin to find out?

2 If I am giving an individual a sedative syrup, what is the reason – is it to control behaviour rather than find out reasons for behaviour?

3 List every stage in getting dressed, right down to buttons. Then assess exactly what aspect(s) of dressing your individual can do alone and where they need help. Add to your list a plan of how you might maintain or even improve their independence.

4 Meaningful Routines

In this chapter we will consider how to balance conflicting needs – the organisation, residents or day care clients and staff – and how to achieve flexible individual care within a group living situation.

CONFLICTING NEEDS

The demands on staff are not always from residents or clients!

- The organisation will expect administrative procedures such as daily record sheets to be carried out.

- Relatives and visitors will have various expectations of what makes a 'good' home or day care centre. A misconception of many people is that, because they are being cared for by professionals, whether in a day centre or in a Home, their relative with dementia will not be at risk.

- Staff, too, expect certain working conditions and also may have strong ideas about what residents or day care clients need.

- Day care might be an objective of the organisation but not seen by staff to be a priority.

It is important therefore that all those involved – residents and day care clients, relatives, staff and other professional groups – understand the purpose and the basic philosophy for day care and residential care.

An understanding of the reasons for day care and what it is intended to achieve will influence the particular working practice. For example, if day care aims to help individuals living in their own homes to retain their self-help skills, so that they can continue to cope, this naturally has implications for what you do.

Similarly, an understanding of the reasons for particular working practices of the Home can go some way to establishing an understandable and consistent place for the residents to live. A residential home is a group living situation, and people with dementia may find this too pressured and over-stimulating. This will affect how private space is organised and how flexible the routines are. The needs of the organisation, the staff and the residents must be balanced in such a way that no one loses sight of the fact that the residents' needs are the most important.

FLEXIBLE ROUTINES

A typical day in any Home will involve set routines such as getting up, washing, dressing, having meals and going to bed. These routines, although necessary, should allow for residents to have their own choices and customs. It is not unusual for people who have worked on shifts or whose job demanded early rising to be up and about at the crack of dawn or, alternatively, later in the morning. For people with dementia these learned habits of a lifetime may be those that persist longest, and therefore are important to tolerate. Mrs Begum, for example, has prayed five times each day all her life. To give her life familiar structure as her dementia progresses, she will need help to continue.

One of the most difficult aspects of working with people with dementia is helping them to be as independent as possible – which often means *not* helping them. For example, it can be very exasperating and wearing to allow them to wash and dress themselves – often very slowly indeed – whilst offering help only when they need it. This is often made even more difficult by tight time schedules, such as at meal times or when the cleaners start their work. Nevertheless, it is very important to support their efforts and maintain their confidence and skills. This applies equally to day care.

It is worth considering when day care support begins. Is it when Mr Hastie or Miss Peacock arrive at the Home or does it begin before they are picked up in the minibus? Effective day care begins in the person's own home, and so the staff member becomes an important link and support over a longer period of time, rather than just for a few hours. An outreach worker is in a good position to encourage the person to use their retained abilities and skills.

In the same way, residents and day care clients can take part in ordinary activities of everyday living. They may, of course, not be interested and should not be forced. Some people have never undertaken household chores and may gain no pleasure from doing them. Most people, though, do have these skills. Generally speaking, women have skills in cooking and cleaning whereas men may prefer do-it-yourself or gardening jobs. Every Home and day centre has domestic chores that need to be done, so there are endless possibilities for working together:

cooking	hoovering
dusting	sweeping
laundering	washing up
ironing	tidying rooms
making beds	going shopping

Sometimes the chores will not be done very well – cups may have to be washed again and table cloths ironed later – but this is not a reason to stop residents taking part. Some Homes have very gifted cooks and cleaners who know exactly how to involve the residents and build their confidence and self-esteem. Other Homes may not have cleaners, which means that staff and residents have to do all the chores. There are some Homes where all the cooking and cleaning are done by staff and residents because the activity and sharing bring such a lot of benefit to everyone. Life in a Home can be very boring if there is nothing to do, and this inactivity leads to a downward spiral of loss of skills, loss of confidence and lost opportunities.

GROUP LIVING BUT INDIVIDUAL CARE

Social relationships are important because they help give a person a feeling of self-worth and value. Ways that you can bring people together for friendships and fun include:

- exercising;
- singing;
- dancing;
- reminiscence groups;
- residents' meetings.

If you are too busy to get a group together, many of these activities can be done as you do your caring duties. For example, you can sing together in the bathroom, dance towards the tea table and reminisce while you help a resident into bed. The person with dementia can still gain some enjoyment from being involved, particularly if for even a short period they experience some pleasure and feeling of being in control.

Typically, residents and day care clients sit in the same chair in the same sitting room with the same group for most of the day. You might like to sit with them in order to be more aware of what goes on. Many lounges have only enough chairs for residents; typically, residents sit and staff stand. Standing is not the best way to tune in to the group's feelings and to discover possible tensions. Neither is it helpful in day care for the staff to be rushing around organising activities, with little time spent sitting with your clients. How would you get round this? Perhaps you could bring in a chair from another room? Or even sit on the floor? Or engage in an activity that involves one-to-one contact seated at a table?

Some people may not be able to talk about what they are thinking and feeling. Facial expression and general demeanour are therefore important indicators about how an individual is feeling. So you need to be more aware of non-verbal communications in sitting rooms even when that individual is not apparently participating. Remember also that our facial expression, manner and body posture can say so much!

You may wonder whether it is worth trying to aim for normal social behaviour in your lounge. When it works well, it can make everyone feel better because they are behaving like ordinary adults. However, a common group problem for people with dementia is that they may not be tolerated by the mentally alert residents. This creates additional pressures for staff as you find yourself continually having to act as a referee and having to respond to the very different demands of the residents:

- People with dementia feel threatened and unsettled, and often do not understand why their behaviour is causing problems.

- The mentally alert residents may feel threatened by the unpredictable behaviour of the person with dementia and the often high emotions being expressed.

- Mentally alert residents might also object to day care clients invading and disrupting their space.

It is important for all residents and day care clients to have private space and a quiet area; no one lives permanently in groups. This is a strong argument for single bedrooms, small sitting areas or quiet places where people can be on their own or with just one or two others. If you have a group of people with dementia who cause a lot of upset to the other residents, it might be worth arranging for a sitting room that is theirs at certain times of the day. It is hard to suggest general guidelines because some people with dementia are much loved by the other residents. Other people with dementia can be so difficult to cope with that you may need to consider having a separate sub-unit for them, everyone mixing only for special occasions.

Individual care

Mrs Amble The staff feel that they do not really know much about Mrs Amble and her past, despite her being in the Home for a month. She has adapted to the Home routine but does not like to leave her bedroom. When staff talk to her she seems to reply as if she were living in the 1950s and refers to a particular staff member as a sister (long since dead). The manager and staff team think they need to know more about her.

One way of finding out more about Mrs Amble would have been to have visited her in her own home before she was admitted. Meeting Mrs Amble in surroundings that were familiar to her would have made it possible to observe how well or poorly she coped with daily living skills. Valuable understanding could have been gained from her immediate surroundings and the significance of her possessions and photographs. These could act as prompts to obtain information about significant events and relationships, so she should be encouraged to bring them with her into the Home.

It is important to begin with the feelings that Mrs Amble might have about herself and her situation and to acknowledge these rather than ignore them.

Talking over the situation with her former home care assistant, Jean, and neighbours would also provide essential information about Mrs Amble.

In planning the continuing care of Mrs Amble, her life history and social background must be considered. A care plan should encourage her to make maximum use of her abilities and to maintain her dignity, respect and self-esteem.

CONTINUITY OF CARE – THE CARE PLAN

Staff should get to know the person with dementia as early as possible so that, as the illness progresses, they can respond in a helpful way. Currently the most usual way is to appoint a 'befriender'. (Sometimes they are called key workers or primary care workers.) If the individual can choose this person, so much the better. It is also important for the befriender to feel positively about the individual.

A care plan can provide all staff with a guide to the individual care required by each person. This will ensure that there is consistency and continuity in the way they are treated. It will also enable staff to avoid stereotyping – to remember that each person is an individual.

Mr Hastie, for example, is known to get angry when he is not busy and active. His care plan has assessed his capacity for certain kinds of activities. He thinks he is at work, and it has been agreed that this is beneficial so all staff must go along with this. He also likes to eat on his own because he is very self-conscious about his chewing problem. This is in the plan and he is always given a special side table where he eats his sandwiches and drinks his flask of tea.

However, any care plan requires that *all* staff:

■ acknowledge the need for continuous regular assessment and adjustment according to the changing needs of the individual;

- are in agreement about how that person can live in the Home or attend day care with the minimum disruption to preferred routines and choices;
- agree to use the person's retained skills and strengths;
- agree on the level of support needed for the person's missing skills.

MEAL TIMES

When and what we eat is another area of life where we all differ. For example, a cooked lunch in the middle of the day may have been the norm for some people, whereas others are used to a cooked evening meal.

Meal times should be planned knowing that people will require varying degrees of help. You need to be able to give that support without the pressure of serving and clearing up at the same time. Noise and bustle in the dining/kitchen area should be kept to a minimum and everyone allowed to dine in a sociable, relaxed setting. All the senses should be tantalised by taste, colour, smell and touch.

You should sit with residents or day care clients, encouraging conversation so that meals are a shared pleasurable experience rather than a routine to be completed as fast as possible. It may be that the more dependent people require a separate dining time. If, for example, someone can no longer manage a knife and fork, can finger food be prepared for them? This is more dignified than someone else cutting up the food and feeding them. Some individuals will need prompting and reminding sometimes, and this is more acceptable if done quietly by someone sitting beside them.

Some people with dementia may not be able to cope with meal times at all and may need to have plates of finger food, such as small sandwiches, slices of fruit and cake, brought to them regularly through the day.

Many people with dementia use food as a means of communication. They might be feeling ill, angry or upset and so refuse their food. By eating with them you will be able to act quickly to deal with the cause of the problem.

OPPORTUNITIES AND RELATIONSHIPS

Throughout a typical day there are many opportunities for all staff to make the person with dementia feel valued. Reminiscing and stimulating activities need not just be a planned event. You can prompt this by sharing and discussing everyday things. For example:

- Accompany a resident or client to the dining room.
- Stop at a window and comment on the view.
- Pick up objects such as ornaments and fruit for the resident or client to hold.
- Get the resident or client to feel the curtains, smell the flowers, pat the dog.

Another way you can make sure that people remember who they are is to use a name for them which they recognise and with which they feel comfortable. Forms of address such as 'Pop', 'Gran' or 'Dear' can be very unhelpful, especially if they have never had any children. These terms also diminish the status of the individuals and can create an atmosphere in which staff do not see the residents or day care clients as adults. Find out how they want to be addressed. Some people will be happy for you to use their first name; others would be offended, though, and would prefer you to be formal – Mr, Mrs or Miss.

Also avoid dehumanising rituals such as handing out tea with milk and sugar already added and tying bibs around people's necks before eating.

PERSONAL HYGIENE

Personal hygiene is a matter that can create embarrassment and distress. Managing continence through the use of aids and toileting regimes is more acceptable if sensitively carried out. A person's dignity is not enhanced by queuing outside toilets after meals or by being publicly summoned to the toilet. Avoid phrases such as '*we* need to go to the toilet'. Remember that it is no more acceptable to be left on a toilet for hours than it is to sit in soiled clothing. Where possible, the individual should be able to choose the gender of the person to deal with their personal hygiene.

It is also good to have someone of the same gender helping with bathing and dressing. Bathing can be a very relaxing and pleasant experience and also offers opportunities for conversations. If bathrooms are warm and full of good smells, a bath can be an activity in itself.

Some people like to bathe daily, others weekly. Some like a shower, whereas others may be frightened of it. Try to find out from your residents which they prefer. Feeling clean and fresh, with clean teeth and fresh clothing can be a great morale booster.

Sometimes people with dementia just forget about the need to wash, and a gentle reminder is all that is needed. In others there may be a reason for their actively refusing to wash or to change into fresh clothes; you will have to try to find out why there is a problem and to work out a solution – which might be just that they don't like the soap's perfume. Day care clients are just as susceptible to neglecting personal cleanliness, especially if they live alone.

Teeth can be neglected. Staff may need to prompt a resident to take dentures out at night for cleaning and to put them in again in the morning. Poorly fitting dentures can be a source of great discomfort and even pain, which the person with dementia may not be able to explain. People who have their own teeth may also need to be reminded. Demonstrating by example may be helpful.

Sometimes it needs imagination and trial and error to achieve results. Mrs Amble, for example, had had dentures for a very long time, but if the care assistant cleaned them and then put them in Mrs Amble's hand she could not remember what to do with them. If, however, the care assistant handed Mrs Amble her teeth with a tooth brush, Mrs Amble brushed her teeth and slipped them into her mouth in one long-familiar movement.

RECORD KEEPING

All this effort requires a lot of organisation. It works best if there is a very clear system of record keeping for everyone, with a carefully worked out care plan and a key worker in charge of each person's case. It is helped if staff meet regularly as a group to share ideas about what is working for an individual and what is not, to report any changes and to share their own concerns and feelings. This sharing is particularly necessary when things are going wrong or caring is becoming stressful. It is also important when everything is going well.

The system of recording and storing care plans should be accessible and user-friendly. The participation of the resident or day care client is essential in formulating the plan; the less the individual is able to take an active part, the more family and friends should become involved. In the absence of these supporters an independent advocate should be appointed to ensure that the person's interests are being maintained.

KEY POINTS

- The requirements of Home or day centre routine and staff practices should never lose sight of the fact that the residents' and clients' needs are the most important.
- Get to know the person with dementia before admission by visiting them in their own home.
- People can be given important stimulating activities if staff encourage involvement in simple daily living tasks.
- Encourage group interactions, but also provide private space and a quiet area.
- Meal times should be a social occasion.
- All opportunities should be used by staff to stimulate and form relationships with the residents and day care clients.
- Care plans are a means for staff to tailor care to the important life events for the individual.
- Day care begins in the person's own home.

TRAINING EXERCISES

1 Mrs Amble has little idea whether it is night or day. She was very anxious and bewildered in her own home and the move into your Home – which was not her decision – has made her even more so. She smokes in bed and this is clearly a fire risk, but it is a lifelong habit so stopping would result in withdrawal symptoms that would cause her great distress. Her habit of walking about at night and trying to leave the Home is upsetting everyone, especially the night staff. How can she be helped?

2 It is good practice to provide activities that build up the confidence and self-esteem of residents or day care clients, and few activities are better than those relating to chores in a kitchen. List the advantages and disadvantages of a kitchen in a unit for people with dementia and the risks that might be taken. How many of these risks can be justified?

5 Dilemmas and Challenges

Provision of group or long-term care is always fraught with dilemmas and challenges: there are no right answers. There are instead ways of facing what is going on and ways of working towards the best possible outcome for all concerned. Dilemmas and challenges are unavoidable in the inevitably artificial business of providing group care, which is seldom what people would choose had there been other options. There is a basic tension always present in providing individual care and care of a group at the same time. This chapter looks first at some of the dilemmas and then at some of the challenges.

DILEMMAS

Conflicts of interest

Conflicts of interest are inevitable in any social situation. It is impossible to provide exactly what one person needs without taking away from someone else. We all compromise to some extent whether we are with one other person or ten but in some group living situations it can seem as if one party is doing all the compromising.

Mr Ho has become very unsettled in the Home, where he has been for one month. No arrangements for his preferences for Chinese food and environment have yet been made because staff are finding it difficult to communicate with him. He is trying to wander out of the Home and continually stands and bangs at the locked door. He becomes extremely angry and walks up and down the lounge shouting in Chinese at the other residents and the day care clients. Some of the care staff are frightened of him, as is Miss Peacock; they feel that he is liable to lash out aggressively towards them or the residents and they want him to be moved.

Conflict of interest between one resident and the group in the Home is a very familiar problem, especially when the individual is someone with challenging behaviour. The usual outcome is the removal of the disruptive individual to another setting or group, which can leave everyone else feeling guilty and less able to cope should it happen again. It is always preferable to try to meet the needs of the individual in such a way that they fit in better.

In *The Lost Ones*, Faith Gibson has described a project in which the most difficult resident in a Home was made the special focus of an attempt to use the past in dealing with their behaviour. Careful life histories were taken, as were very detailed notes of the person's preferences to see if staff in the Home could communicate with the resident and understand the behaviour better. In some cases this was very successful. This approach might well work with Mr Ho: he is likely to have very particular preferences which will not be obvious to care staff unless they have a Chinese background similar to that of Mr Ho.

Conflicts of interest between residents or day care clients

A very familiar result of this conflict of interests is when a routine is changed to meet the needs of an individual and everyone suffers. A locked door might preserve one person's safety but it would diminish the quality of life of the others. This is a very familiar pattern in residential and nursing homes. Once again the answer is to look at the needs of the individual.

- Do they need more exercise? Perhaps they could take part in dancing, exercise sessions or walks?
- Are they bored? Find out what they enjoy doing.
- Are they feeling insecure and searching for a familiar place? Try to find ways to make them feel more settled.

In a Home, try to find ways of making it more 'familiar' by using the resident's own possessions and their choice of pictures and so on. You may find that some people are anxious and insecure at certain times of the day and will need some extra attention or activity until this passes.

Conflicts of interest between staff and residents or day care clients

Conflicts of interest between the staff and the residents or day care clients are also very common. The staff, for example, may find it easier to cope with a very restless person who has been sedated. Staff may prefer locked doors because it means they do not have to be on the alert all the time. Staff may like to do the washing up because it gets it done more quickly. Day care centres may find that their willing volunteers like to be involved in practical ways, and so often stifle the person's motivation to help themselves.

Another, often neglected, issue is the decor of a Home or centre. Who decides and on what basis? Most usually it is the staff who choose the wallpaper and paint. It is staff who choose the pictures. It is staff who like the place to be tidy. It is staff who choose not to put individual signs on the doors. Sometimes they are trying to meet the needs of the relatives who like to see an attractive and tidy place. But in fact it is the residents or day care clients who spend the most time there and their wishes are more important.

Conflicts of interest with relatives

Another area of conflict of interests is that between the relatives and the person with dementia. This relationship can be full of unresolved emotion when a relative has, in effect, put the person with dementia into long-term care. They need to feel that the person with dementia is as safe as, or safer than, they were at home and is as well if not better cared for than they were at home. This is particularly the case when balancing rights and risk, discussed in the next section.

The mixed feelings of relatives can sometimes mean that they seem to complain a lot. It is well worth spending time with them, letting them voice their sadness and feelings of guilt. You can then have a more constructive discussion about what is best for the individual.

Relatives may, however, be less unselfish and not want to spend money on the person with dementia so will not be willing to contribute to outings, clothes or whatever is required for that individual. Often extra spending is, in effect, spending their inheritance.

You may sometimes find yourself in a very difficult position between relatives and residents or day care clients. It might be helpful then to set up a formal meeting, with someone there to speak on behalf of the individual. It is certainly not always appropriate to accept the decision of the relative. You may need to contact the social worker to consider legal action if you feel that a resident or day care client's money is being mismanaged or an individual is being abused in some way.

Rights and risk

The matter of rights and risk is basically about the balance between the duty to protect and the liberty of the resident or day care client as an adult with the same rights as anyone else. It is a very difficult line to tread, especially with people with dementia who have difficulties with understanding, memory and reasoning.

The locked door is perhaps the clearest expression of this principle. You may feel uneasy about actually locking a door but not be too concerned about a door with two handles or buttons to press. But for the person with dementia, the door is locked because they cannot open it. This can make them anxious or angry, so they shake the door all day long.

As with all matters of risk, it is important to weigh up the alternatives. Is it possible to leave the door open and have a safe, attractive garden? Is it possible to give your energetic 'escapees' more exercise or to accompany them when they want to go out?

Part of this complex issue is the role of the family. They cannot legally speak on behalf of the person with dementia yet clearly they do all the time. If they do not like the care their relative is getting, they can move them or constantly complain. This can be very difficult because the better Homes and day centres will have a philosophy of allowing residents and day care clients as much liberty to do what they want within the bounds of responsible care. The family and the manager may have quite different ideas about where the line is drawn.

A family member may go to the Registration or Inspection service with their complaint which will then be investigated. If your Home or day centre has clear policies that are being implemented as well as possible, then all that may happen is a clarification of expectations all round. Remember that family members may be feeling guilty at not being able to care for their relative and may therefore be a little unreasonable. You may find that helping them to talk about their feelings clears the air. You may also find that if they can be actively involved in caring for their relative, and sometimes other residents or day care clients too, they will feel less guilty.

Perhaps rights and risk can have too high a profile. They are certainly not the main theme of this book. We have emphasised the more important considerations of dignity, privacy and making the most of the potential of the failing brain and personality. An over-preoccupation with rights and risk can endanger these more important but closely related aspects of care. Fire regulations, for example, can be interpreted very fiercely, resulting in a limitation on the freedom of people with dementia who may not be able to open a heavy door or who may want to use a kitchen that has to be behind walls rather than a counter.

We are not helped by the way that society deals with this dilemma. Legislation is invariably in the direction of limiting risk, whatever the implications for quality of life. One of the difficulties facing staff on this issue is the mass media's attitude that any suggestion that one should be less than 100 per cent zealous in protecting residents or day care clients from harm is interpreted as carelessness. It is much easier for the ill-informed public to be scandalised by someone in residential or day care being hurt or killed when doing what the rest of us do daily than it is for them to be scandalised by the restrictions and poor quality of life that elimination of all risk promotes.

Some local authorities have faced up to this problem by clearly stating in all written material about their Homes and day care centres that residents or clients are encouraged to be as independent as possible and that there may be some risks involved. They explain that people with dementia need to be allowed to do as much as they can do safely if they are to retain their skills and confidence. Some private and voluntary Homes also state this. It is a great help to staff if they know that they will not be blamed if someone in their care gets hurt.

Sadly, there seems at present to be a tide flowing the other way, with constant discussion of tagging, video cameras and passive alarm systems.

Restricting activity

Tagging is where an electronic device is worn by the residents, so that staff will know when they have gone through certain doors. Video cameras can be located in corridors and hallways. Passive alarm systems are those that record the footsteps of residents – usually by the bed or the bathroom door. These devices are sometimes seen as a substitute for staff. They really should not be necessary if the unit is run in such a way that the residents' habits and preferences are well known and there are good care regimes.

Counsel and Care have produced a booklet on restraint, *What If They Hurt Themselves?*, designed to encourage discussion and offer some sensible approaches. They describe the Buxton chair, which is a tipping chair that totally immobilises the person, and is rarely seen in reputable units. Chairs with very restricting tables are seen more often and the use of medicines or drugs is probably more common than we like to imagine. Interestingly, in the USA where residents are eight times more likely to be physically restrained, they are also twice as likely to fall and break a limb. There are many paradoxes in this world of dilemmas. Sometimes leaving a gate open stops people trying to leave.

It is in this area of restraint that guidance has been developed on setting the limits for such action. The Royal College of Nursing, for example, has guidelines which suggest that:

- Such a decision should always be made by the team providing care.
- It should always be recorded and a time limit set.
- If it is continued, it should be thoroughly reviewed at regular intervals.

This set of steps should apply to any action that diminishes the quality of life of someone who is unable to understand what is happening and who cannot speak out on their own behalf.

To mix or not to mix?

A group made up of similar people will be more relaxed, feel safer and will promote harmony whereas a mixed group will be more vigorous and exciting and potentially stressful. There are advantages and disadvantages for both types. There is, once again, no right answer.

Here the dilemma at its most basic is whether or not to mix people with dementia with people who are mentally alert. At a more subtle level the next dilemma is whether to mix people with dementia who have behaviour problems with those who are relatively well adjusted; or whether to mix those in the terminal stages with those who are still active.

In specialist units for people with dementia, the dilemma is whether to mix people with high levels of challenging behaviour, people who are calm in their dementia and people who are dying. Most places mix all three without really thinking about it. This is in part because they do not know how to make a distinction.

There are some useful 'dependency scales', such as the Extended Crichton Behaviour Rating Scale (see Appendix 2), which can be very helpful in looking objectively at the different kinds of dependency in your residents or day care clients. You may need to ask a psychologist in your local psychiatric hospital to advise you about the scales. By comparing the results, you may find that there is a match between groups of residents or day care clients, which means that you can tailor your regime to suit their needs. This is often not possible because of limitations of space, but it is worth thinking about.

Related to the 'mix' issue is whether to mix people in day and long-stay care, or to mix people in respite and long-stay care. Recent research by Ann Netten suggests that a constant change of residents makes permanent residents with dementia more disorientated.

There are no right answers with any of these dilemmas; there are only right questions. Whose needs are being met? What is the best possible outcome for *all* participants, including staff and relatives? Has a fair compromise been achieved and communicated to all concerned?

If we apply these questions to the dilemma of mix we might get the following answers.

Mixing mentally alert people with dementia sufferers might meet the needs of the alert. If alert residents or day care clients are worried that they will develop dementia, they will be very anxious that they may be treated as less than a full member of the community. If they have seen other people being treated with respect and helped to cope with their dementia, though, they are less likely to be fearful and more likely to ask for help.

Mixing the two groups might meet the needs of those with dementia who then get the stimulation of mentally alert people. It might also meet the interests of the staff because they will not be weighed down by a group who are all very mentally dependent. And it might meet the interests of some of the family who may not want to face the fact that their relative has dementia. On the other hand, alert people can be very distressed by mixing with those with dementia. People with dementia can be abused by alert and exasperated people. Staff may prefer to concentrate on the special needs of people with dementia. Relatives may want specialist care.

Each of these considerations needs to be weighed up for the particular setting in relation to what alternatives exist and the particular circumstances. For example, a new resident might relax in the residential setting and be a very pleasant addition to the Home. They might be well known to the other residents if they were local people, and other residents might be pleased to have the newcomer among them even with a failing brain. On the other hand, the same person might be very sour and angry. They might shout all the time that they wanted to go home and they might constantly go into the wrong room at all times of the day and night. In these circumstances they might well be better cared for by staff who are used to managing difficult behaviour and in a small group where their behaviour is less upsetting to the others.

Exactly the same question applies to the mixing of day care clients and respite people with permanent residents. The residents may find day and respite people very disruptive, given the difficulties they have with remembering new people. On the other hand, day and respite people may benefit from learning gradually about the setting into which they will finally be placed. Staff, too, may enjoy the coming and going of less disabled people, to relieve the tedium of caring for people who are very dependent. Relatives of those in long-stay care may have different views from those whose family member is receiving day or respite care.

Once again, the key is to be clear about whose needs are being met and to work towards a compromise that meets the maximum.

Cost and staffing are always issues, and sometimes not much can be done about either. These are key issues and need to be out in the open. Sometimes people pretend that they have made decisions on the basis of what is best for the individual when in fact costs and staffing were the real reasons. Being clear about the reason for things promotes problem-solving attitudes and the seizing of opportunities when they arise. If, for example, you are clear that the reason you cannot use a particular lounge for day people is that you cannot afford tables and chairs for lunch times, you can put the problem to the local Rotary club when they visit your Home and ask for their help in solving it.

CHALLENGES

Sex

Sex is a challenge in long-term care. Just because someone may have dementia does not mean that they will not have sexual needs and feelings. Such feelings are likely to go unnoticed unless the individual begins to behave in ways that challenge our attitudes and thinking about what we consider to be acceptable behaviour. How you respond is based on the following three important issues.

1 Open expression

This relates to the ways in which the sexuality and sexual needs of a person are acknowledged. For instance, does your Home or day care centre encourage open demonstration of affection? Hugs, cuddles and holding hands can often alleviate anxiety.

2 Challenging behaviour

Some people with dementia behave in a sexually disinhibited fashion. They may masturbate in public or make advances to others in a sexually explicit way. You must be able to make a calm appraisal of the reasons for such behaviour. Being able to talk sensibly about what has happened is good staff practice and prevents damaging over-reaction.

3 Acknowledge the past

Some individuals may have been the subject of sexual abuse and violence, so their view of 'normal' sexuality is dramatically different.

The three main questions that you should consider are:

- How do you meet the sexual needs of your residents?

- How do you deal with deviant sexual behaviour?
- How do you deal with the legacy of sexual abuse from the past?

There may be a problem because of people's reluctance to talk about sex, often because they do not have the language. It is crucial that the manager takes the lead in making this a topic of easy discussion so that staff learn how to talk about it. You may have to decide what words are appropriate; generally the more straightforward terminology is best. Some members of staff may have particular difficulty talking about homosexual sex and a firm lead may be needed to prevent embarrassed giggles or the use of language such as 'poofter' or 'fairy'.

Mrs Amble is constantly going into the rooms of two of the male residents and indicating that she wants to have sex with them. One is keen and the other is plainly alarmed. The staff are at a loss to know what to do for the best and their initial reaction is to chase Mrs Amble out of the rooms with a ticking off. The other residents are aware that something uncomfortable is going on. Mrs Amble's former home care assistant, Jean, who is a regular visitor, is aghast and says that Mrs Amble's behaviour is an insult to the memory of her dead husband. She wants staff to lock the door of Mrs Amble's bedroom.

Mrs Amble clearly needs some sexual contact and it would seem that one of the men would welcome this. Given the inability of people with dementia to make their wishes known clearly, staff need good skills of communication. In order to look clearly at such a situation, staff need to have a lead from the manager in terms of how it is talked about and the language used. Jean also needs help in talking the situation through and considering whose needs are being met by her attitude. The needs of the other residents are for a calm, well ordered house, so a resolution of this issue will be a priority.

There will be a compromise solution which goes some way to meeting the needs of *all* parties but it will take very careful work to achieve it. It may be necessary for members of staff to speak on behalf of Mrs Amble and the two men, assuming that they have dementia and are not able to speak for themselves. Once the solution has been arrived at, all parties (including all relevant staff) will need to know so that everyone acts appropriately and according to the agreement.

Mrs Amble is a woman who has had a full life, during which time she has had preferences and opportunities for making choices. As far as possible she should go on making choices; if she cannot communicate them, an attempt should be made to make them on the lines she would have in the past. In this case Jean is trying to make a choice on her behalf which is very difficult and legally not really appropriate. It is probably not safe to assume that Jean knows much about Mrs Amble's attitudes to sex.

Suppose that the decision is made to lock Mrs Amble's door at night because both men do not welcome her advances and she does not respond to explanations. This decision must be written down together with the names of those who made the decision, the reasons given and a short timetable set for review. Decisions do occasionally have to be made to restrain people but this should be a last resort and rigid safeguards are required.

In any long-stay setting the whole group of residents and staff form a living entity whose welfare and happiness are crucial. A tradition of talking openly about issues of concern will make dealing with this sort of problem much easier. Pushing it 'under the carpet' may only lead to petty vindictiveness and nasty gossip. There are group norms of behaviour in any group setting and the tone is invariably set by the strongest person: the good manager will make sure that it is them.

Spiritual needs

Very different but equally neglected are spiritual needs. Many Homes have an occasional religious service. Few, though, offer opportunities for quiet reflection or prayer; yet these very familiar, long-standing traditions may be very important indeed to the person with dementia who is unable to express what they are missing.

People often have strong views and preferences regarding religion, and these are not always predictable. It is not enough to know a person's religion. You need to know if regular attendance at a place of worship is important, and so arrangements should be made for a resident to be taken, or if a minister of the appropriate religion could visit the Home or day care centre. Also find out if they like to pray at certain times of the day, if they like to pray alone or with others, if they need a shrine, and so on. Mrs Begum, for example, needs to pray at times set by the local mosque. Be careful not to assume that people who do not attend religious services do not have spiritual needs: it may be music or nature, but there is probably something they need in order to feel at peace.

Ethnic minorities

Dementia in people from ethnic minority communities is a real challenge both to people providing care for older people from ethnic minorities and to those providing care for people with dementia. Neither group has addressed this issue adequately. Yet it is crucially important to provide care that is culturally appropriate. People with dementia will not easily adjust to the unfamiliar and may have forgotten recently learned languages and traditions. Both Mr Ho and Mrs Begum illustrate the importance of being sensitive to different cultures.

Early-onset dementia

Finally, there is an emerging challenge from the new groups of people with early-onset dementia. These include people with Down's syndrome, AIDS, Korsakoff's syndrome, early Alzheimer's disease and early multi-infarct dementia. These are younger people for whom there are few specialist services and who do not fit into the existing services.

As with all the other challenges, we need to face the issue, ask whose needs are being met by the present arrangements, see if we can make changes to meet more people's needs and ensure that the eventual compromise is seen as fair and is communicated to all concerned.

KEY POINTS

- Stop and face the issue.

- Look clearly at what is going on and always ask 'Whose needs are being met?'

- A compromise solution will have to be seen as fair by all parties, and will have to be effectively communicated, for it to be carried out.

- Remember that everyone is an individual with a history and that the group is a living entity too.

- Any decision that diminishes the quality of life of the weakest party (ie the residents or day care clients) should be regularly reviewed.

TRAINING EXERCISE

1   What would you do with a resident like Mrs Amble who was making advances to male residents? Do you find that you are shocked that a woman is behaving like this?

2   What do you think are the ethical issues to be considered when thinking of using passive alarm systems?

6 Good Design

Good design does not make good things happen – it makes them possible.

Most people are not consciously aware of the impact of design on their lives except at extremes such as a leaking roof or a squeaky door. Most of us, however, have feelings about buildings. We like to be in some and dislike others, without really analysing why. This chapter aims to make you more aware of the built environment and the effect it has on people with dementia and the staff who care for them.

There are important principles, based on a general agreement of opinion from research and from people working in specialist care of people with dementia, which can be considered.

- A building should make sense.
- A building should help people find their way around.
- A building should provide a therapeutic environment.
- A building should provide a safe environment.
- A building should minimise staff stress.

A building should make sense

For most people a domestic, or home-like, environment is the most familiar.

Many residents and day care clients with dementia think they are in:

- a hotel
- a hospital

- a workplace

because they cannot explain the environment in any other terms that make sense to them.

The Home or day care centre may not resemble anywhere that the person with dementia has been before. This may determine their behaviour, especially in the sense that they will want to leave to go home.

People with dementia are less able to work things out and have a very poor memory. Buildings therefore need to have an obviousness about them. In practice this is very difficult because group living is not a familiar experience for most people.

Some large old houses, having once been domestic homes, do have a familiar logic to them in the sense that public rooms are generally on the ground floor, toilets are generally at the back of the building and there is usually a hall from which there are doors to the main rooms. This familiar logic will probably not be as familiar to Mr Ho and Mrs Begum. It would be interesting for staff to ask the families where they lived as children and young adults. Staff might then appreciate why Mr Ho and Mrs Begum are not always able to find their way around the Home.

Size

Making an establishment for large numbers of people seem homely is not easy. Size is a key factor for obvious reasons.

Because people with dementia often cannot learn new things easily, they can only be expected to get to know a few people and in as small a space as possible. There is no evidence about what size is best: eight is the number that is most often quoted but this is surprising really, considering that very few of us have lived our lives in groups as big as eight; indeed, if eight residents in a Home means having eight staff, we are talking about a group of sixteen. It is possible, though, to design new units that are relatively homely with eight people. A building in a familiar locality will also have more chance of making sense.

Adapting an existing building

How can you adapt your present building to make sense to someone with dementia? Sub-units need to be as homely as possible. The rest of the building is less important because most people will stay in their sub-unit.

Making corridors look like streets or landings may be more useful than making them look homely, because houses and flats rarely have corridors in them.

A Home in Glasgow has decided that their corridor is not at all homely and is best painted to look like a landing in an old-fashioned tenement. All the bedroom doors look like flat doors and there is even a gas light. They claim that this makes sense to many of their residents. Are there any changes that could be made in your Home or day care centre?

Furniture and fittings

Consider using traditional furniture and light fittings. Fireplaces were a feature of all houses until recently and can make a homely focus for a room. A completely artificial fireplace may add to confusion because it will not give off any heat; this may or may not matter to your group of residents or day care clients. If they are willing, it can be helpful to have residents' possessions in the public areas so that they feel more familiar.

A building should help people find their way around

Staff caring for people with dementia spend a lot of time escorting them to where they need to be:

- to the toilet;
- to their bedroom;
- to the public rooms.

Staff usually say that this is because people with dementia cannot find their way. The person with dementia therefore becomes dependent on the staff, with the result that they lose their independence and dignity. With appropriate cues, however, it should be possible for some of the residents or day care clients to find their own way.

Toilets

Toilets are the most important place to find. Unfortunately, many build-ings make this difficult because:

- toilets are out of sight of the living areas;
- most door signs are too high and too modern.

Even when standing by the toilet door, the person with dementia would often have to be tall and able to read and understand either the word 'toilet' or the modern matchstick-person symbol.

In an existing building the answer to the toilet door problem is to make it different. In *People with Dementia*, Faith Gibson describes how Ferrard House let residents choose between samples of colours and discovered that they could differentiate a plum colour. Now all their toilet doors are plum coloured, which makes them very different from other doors. Some Homes and day care centres have chosen yellow, others a bright red. These places recognise that the ability to tell one colour from another diminishes with age but remains best in the red/yellow area of the spectrum.

Some Homes or day care centres have chosen to put a picture of an old-fashioned toilet on the door. It may not be attractive to have a picture of a toilet on the door, but, before finally deciding, watch the residents or clients to see whether it works. If it does, giving them some indepen-dence may make it worth having a possibly distasteful sign. All of the Homes with colours and signs claim that they have enabled some of the residents to find their own way. What cues are there in your Home or day care centre?

Bedrooms

Residents' bedrooms are another key place but few Homes have any guide to finding them. All the doors look the same except for a number or sometimes a small name plate.

How does your Home deal with this problem? Remember that residents are individuals and no one system will help all of them. For example:

- some will remember a number;
- others will be able to read their name;
- some will recognise a photograph;

- others need a solid object such as a plant or a door knocker;

- others will recognise a picture of a favourite place or hobby.

The answer is to try different ideas. In Ferrard House many residents think that the photographs on their doors (neatly protected by a simple 6 × 3 inch wood and Perspex holder) are actually of their mother or father but some are able to recognise it. In *Pink Doors and Door Knockers*, Nicholas Bell describes how, in Rosebank, which has many cues such as name, number, photograph and door knocker, many residents can manage at least one of the cues.

Sitting rooms and dining rooms

These rooms are often behind closed doors; even when the doors are open, this gives little indication about what goes on in the rooms so that the individual is prepared. Some residential homes and day care centres do not have a separate dining room, others simply have tables with no indication of what happens. Residents or day care clients may have their meals at a table that earlier had been used for craft work or games. This situation adds to the disorientation of a person with dementia.

Some ideas that you can consider are:

- Careful positioning of plants, pictures and hangings can make it easier for people to recognise certain corridors, hall ways and dining rooms.

- Living area doors should have panes of glass in them so that people can see what the room is. This can be done whether you are adapting an existing building or building new.

- Good lighting is vital in helping people to find their way round.

- Related to good lighting is the importance of having non-reflecting flooring. People with dementia often think that shiny floors are pools of water and are fearful of walking on them independently.

When planning a new wing or unit, there is the opportunity to make all doors visible from everywhere in the unit. Toilets ought to be visible from the living areas and from the beds. Ideally, and this is a design challenge that few have overcome, rooms should all be off the living area so that, wherever the individual is, they can see where they want to be. If you were planning a new unit, how would you try to achieve this?

A building should provide a therapeutic environment

A therapeutic environment is one that:

- Enables the person with dementia to function at the highest possible level.

- Provides opportunities for purposeful activity, so it will have a real kitchen for doing real jobs such as washing up and a workbench so that men can do woodwork. It may also have a garden with a greenhouse or raised beds and a domestic-scale laundry.

- Reduces the uncertainty and fear that are the disabling consequences of dementia.

- Provides enough but not too much stimulation. Thus it will be a quiet environment with only meaningful sounds. There will be places and windows from which individuals can watch without joining in – an activity that some people enjoy in most Homes.

- Reinforces individual identity because people with dementia need constant reminders about who they are. In a Home, single rooms let unfurnished are the best way of achieving this because the room is then likely to be full of the resident's own possessions.

Mr Hastie Some of the staff were finding it difficult to cope with Mr Hastie. He did not enjoy the activities that were available and was unwilling to take part. Instead, he followed staff around all the time, telling them that the walls needed rebuilding.

The answer to Mr Hastie's restless and demanding behaviour was found in his do-it-yourself talents. He can be kept happily occupied at the workbench, fixing furniture. In the summer he is especially pleased to be outside in the garden shed. He likes to paint it and generally keep it ship-shape. These activities make sense to him as an ex-builder.

Cost constraints

There are always cost constraints, but the right environment is as therapeutic as medicines or activities or even staff. Carpets are a good example. Whether and where to have carpets is debated as if it were about good practice but it is often about cost savings. Given the right equipment and staff training, they should be less effort to keep clean than vinyl which requires wiping and then polishing. Generally speaking, they are therapeutic because they make the place feel homely and they soak up noise. Thus they are a therapeutic priority even if they have to be replaced after a while. Clearly, carpets have to be the type that can be easily cleaned because incontinence is likely to be commonplace. In some places, such as beside some beds, an additional rubber-backed mat may be required. However, there are times when a carpet is not a good idea: some people may never have had a fitted carpet in their lives and are much more at home with linoleum and a mat.

Another example is plastic chairs. Staff with a feel for what looks domestic will choose chairs with washable cotton covers over waterproof cushions. These are also less sticky than plastic chairs to sit on for long periods. There are some excellent chintz-covered chairs on the market designed for people with incontinence. Having enough chairs for visitors and staff as well as residents or day care clients is important, as is having a variety of styles. People with dementia need all the clues possible to remind them which is the chair in which they feel comfortable. None of this need cost a lot: it is about understanding the principles and using your imagination.

Adapting an existing building

When adapting an existing building, it can be difficult to provide places where purposeful activity can take place. For example, kitchens are seldom in the right place for people to join in; however, sometimes there are sinks that can be used for washing up. Some people like a conservatory with plants to water or a tool shed.

In Walker House they have adapted a room to be an old-fashioned cafe. In Abbotsford a sink in the corner of the sitting room is used by residents to wash up and then put away the china. Have you been able to make such an adaptation in your Home or centre? Or is there perhaps something that could be changed now?

Being able to sit and watch without having to understand sufficiently to respond is clearly an activity enjoyed by many people with dementia. A large foyer and low window sills with a busy view are much appreciated. Activities such as games and crafts are of course important and there should be space where these can take place.

Single rooms will not be the norm in most Homes in older buildings but much can be done to create individual space. Bellsdyke Hospital is a big, old-fashioned place which has divided its large wards with high room dividers that incorporate chests of drawers and wardrobes. Within this private space residents can keep personal possessions such as pictures and ornaments.

New buildings

Good design in a new building is much easier. Kitchen counters at the end of the living rooms or complete kitchens seen through large hatches become a real possibility, as do sheds and conservatories.

Controlling stimulation is possible in any building up to a point, although it is only in a new building that the traffic of constant deliveries can be kept separate. Carpets are a magic way of reducing confusing noise as well as making places feel more homely (see above). The same applies to curtains and soft furnishings.

Buildings should provide a safe environment

People with dementia are often unable to understand the consequences of their own behaviour. The behaviour that causes most anxiety is what is referred to as 'wandering'. If you watch someone 'wandering', they are often:

- looking for something;
- trying to get out;
- actively taking exercise;
- clearly lost.

Anxieties about people leaving and coming to grief are understandable. But we must try to balance the possible risks involved in someone wandering off with the right to freedom of movement. One officer in charge stopped people 'escaping' over the fence by leaving the gate open! Making buildings make sense so that people do not get lost, and providing plenty of space and plenty of diverting activities are clearly going to help.

'Racetrack' designs around a courtyard or round internal corridors are not helpful for staff or for residents or day care clients. The sight of people going round and round remorselessly is very wearisome for everybody. A circuit through furniture and, if possible, round flowerbeds in the garden is infinitely preferable and affords opportunities to stop and do something else. A recent book about long-stay care, *Special Needs Dementia Units*, maintains that good design and an engaging regime will put an end to wandering.

Outdoors

Safe outdoor space must be a good idea for very active people. It can be designed so it is not an invitation to leave. For example, a straight path to a gate or onto a main road will lead disorientated people clearly in that direction, but a winding path may well take them past something that will distract them because they are not always heading for the gate, they are just following the path.

Gardens should look inwards, with plenty of distractions and thick planting obscuring the fence. An oppressive fence is no less oppressive to a person with dementia; indeed, it may be more so because they do not understand why they are where they are.

Indoors

Concealed plugs, safety radiators and thermostatic showers are now customary.

It is a good idea to attempt to conceal rooms that you do not want the residents or day care clients to enter. The doors can be 'painted out' by making them the same colour as the wall. However, people with only mild dementia might be further confused by seeing staff apparently entering and leaving through a wall, so this may not always be sensible. Cupboards or plants may be a better way of concealing a door.

When planning new buildings, doors that are not for resident or client access should be 'hidden' as far as possible.

Fire regulations are a headache. Invariably, fire doors are at the end of corridors, ensuring that a person with dementia is guided straight through them and out. They can be made less obviously a door and more like a window in some cases, although a clear exit sign is essential. If you are designing from scratch, you will be able to put them into rooms so that they are not in such a direct line.

A building should minimise stress for staff

Face-to-face care for people with dementia is incredibly draining. They demand a level of emotional input and a degree of personal energy that is utterly exhausting. Staff must have somewhere to go and laugh or cry in private. It must be away from the unit, where the residents or clients cannot follow. Separate rooms for the office and for meetings are also essential. If you are a manager and do not want to confuse the people in your care but do want to make the best of your staff, the staff have to participate fully in the life of the unit.

This is easier said than done in many existing buildings with their nurses' stations and their staff rooms just off units. Sometimes rooms can be found in attics or basements. A new unit provides an opportunity to get this right.

KEY POINTS

- Buildings should be as homely as possible.
- Given the right cues, people with dementia may be able to find their way around.
- An environment should provide opportunities for purposeful activity.
- Safe outdoor space should be created.
- Staff should have their own, separate, space.

TRAINING EXERCISES

1   Step into your front hall, and imagine that your reality is the 1940s. What does your front hall remind you of? Could you guess which way to go if you wanted the bedrooms or the main sitting room?

2   Sit in the main living room for a couple of hours with a notebook and record the extent to which it encourages purposeful activity and the amount of potentially helpful 'stimulation' it contains.

7 Health Matters

In this chapter we will consider the illnesses or health problems that may make life for the person with dementia more difficult, and look at ways to prevent or cure them. It is often very helpful to have a doctor who is familiar with the special problems of older people with dementia. But some residents may feel more comfortable with their own GP and their right to choose should be respected.

Day care staff may have to develop close links with the general practitioners of those attending day care. Some day centres have a regular call from a liaison health visitor who can give advice on medication and diet, and generally be kept up to date on the person's health and well-being.

Staff who work in day or residential care are in a unique position because they can observe changes in the person's functioning. When an individual's confusional state suddenly gets worse, it is important to suspect a physical cause and to ask the relative to telephone their doctor.

DEMENTIA: A FATAL ILLNESS

Dementia is a medical condition, and a very serious one at that. At first the person's brain and its workings are affected to only a mild extent, but later more and more brain functions are lost. In the middle stages of dementia, physical signs of the illness begin to appear:

■ Many people will begin to lose control of their bladder and become incontinent of urine, first at night and then all the time.

- Weight loss (or sometimes weight gain) may occur, because the disease process in the brain affects those areas that control our appetite and weight.
- Signs of muscular weakness, stiffness or shakiness become apparent.

Later on these effects become much worse. The individual can become incontinent of both urine and faeces, lose their muscular strength and coordination and become chair- or bed-bound. Epileptic fits can also occur. Eventually the body's defences against disease seem to be affected, so the person is prone to infections such as pneumonia. In the end, death is a result of the dementia, although it may take ten or even fifteen years to reach this very final stage.

Knowing that dementia is not just loss of memory but a fatal illness can lead to the dangerous assumption that any physical illness or disability is directly caused by the dementia, and so can be ignored.

Doing this could mean that people in your centre or Home would be put through quite unnecessary distress. It could mean that they would become disturbed because they feel ill but do not understand what is going on. People with dementia may not be so good as the rest of us at telling where a pain is coming from, or may forget some of their symptoms, or may not be able to communicate their distress (and we are not always very good at these things either). So we have to be on a special lookout for any hints that a person with dementia is also physically ill.

DEMENTIA AND DELIRIUM

One particular sign of illness that is very common among dementia sufferers is called delirium or acute confusion. ('Acute' in medicine means quick.) What happens is that whatever disorder the person is suffering from (an infection, heart failure, unwanted (side) effects of a medicine) affects the workings of the brain temporarily, making them more dopey and muddled, more disorientated, perhaps even to start seeing things that are not there – visual hallucinations. They may get restless and their sleep is likely to be disturbed.

All these things can happen in dementia. But if there is a quick change, and the dementia sufferer rapidly becomes more confused, or develops hallucinations, or gets very sleepy, you should immediately think that there may be a delirium. The doctor should be called and told about the change. He or she may need to be persuaded quite firmly that you think this is delirium, because a doctor who does not see the patient every day may not be very impressed by a change that is obvious to you. To make matters worse, the state of delirium is very variable and it may be that, when the doctor calls, the individual seems to be no different from usual. Sometimes the signs of delirium are very subtle and it is difficult to be sure. Sometimes the change in the person is a change in behaviour, becoming more restless, or becoming aggressive out of the blue, or getting easily upset.

The best advice is always to suspect physical illness when there is any sudden change in a resident or day care client. Indeed, it is a good idea to have regular (say, six-monthly) checks of a person's health, in case important disorders are being missed.

TEN COMMON HEALTH ISSUES

1 Diet and eating

In general, people who suffer from dementia will want to go on eating their usual diet, and keep their usual tastes and preferences. Part of our assessment of a new resident or day care client will include careful gathering of information about this aspect of their lives. However, dementia may bring changes. Some people:

- develop particular likes and dislikes;
- want to eat less;
- eat any (or anybody's) food;
- seem to eat a lot but lose weight;
- gain weight and become obese.

Sometimes several small meals through the day are better than a few bigger meals. Some people prefer to eat smaller meals all the time. Finger food can be helpful for this kind of person.

You should ensure that everyone eats a good balanced diet, paying very particular attention to the need for roughage (fibre) and fluids because constipation is a common problem. If an individual's wish for food changes greatly, or if they seem to be losing weight, even if we think this is due to their dementia, they should have a proper medical check. Conditions such as cancer, diabetes and infections are very common in older people and dementia sufferers are no exception. Difficulty with eating may be caused by a problem with teeth or dentures.

2 Exercise

People with dementia gradually lose their interest in themselves and in what is going on around them. Eventually they become physically weaker; throughout the dementia they may also tend to drop out of social activities. For all these reasons, residents or day care clients (if they are not agitated or restless for some reason) may tend to sit around all day and become physically weaker because of lack of exercise. The danger is that, because they seem to be fairly contented and they are not bothering us, we leave them to sit.

But this will not do. Older people who do not exercise will quickly lose the strength in their muscles. Because of this they will become unsteady and weak on their feet, with the danger of falls or of becoming chair-bound. Once they are sitting around for long periods, they are more prone to pressure sores – with all the discomfort and distress that these cause. Gentle but regular exercise is not only vital to maintain health, it is also good fun and improves the morale of residents or clients and staff alike. Relatives can be involved, too. Dances, walking outings, swimming trips and exercise games are all helpful. And there is some evidence that exercise may actually prevent restlessness.

People with arthritis or who are physically handicapped in some other way can be encouraged to exercise as much as possible while sitting down. Moving to music can be very enjoyable.

3 Alcohol

Occasionally, alcohol has been the cause of a dementia, or of the sort of forgetfulness that is called Korsakoff's syndrome. In these cases the individual should be strongly advised to stop drinking altogether, and specialist help should be sought if necessary. Stopping taking alcohol can actually lead to improvement in the person's memory and general physical health.

However, for others, who have always had a social drink and who happen to suffer from Alzheimer's disease, alcohol does not necessarily do any harm. In a few cases you may find that the person is made more muddled or is more unsteady on their feet after drinking, and here you should advise them to cut down their drinking. Sometimes they may be drinking too much merely because they forget that they have already had one. You can help by keeping alcohol out of their sight.

In a very few cases, dementia actually leads a previously modest drinker into a real alcohol problem. Here you should try to intervene and get control over their drinking. But for most people with dementia continuing their usual level of alcohol intake causes no problems. Indeed, many simply stop drinking when they enter care homes or hospitals.

What we must avoid completely is the old-fashioned practice of using alcohol as a sedative for people who are restless. Alcohol is not only an addictive drug, it is also a dangerous drug with many unwanted effects. As we get older our bodies do not handle alcohol as well as when we were younger, and to start giving someone alcohol late in their life is most unwise.

4 Smoking

There are some people who believe that smoking may improve the circulation to the brain, or even that it could prevent dementia. Doctors more and more, though, see smoking as a curse, which has many, many serious health consequences, and not only lung cancer. It can lead to other cancers, chest problems and poor circulation, and is connected with heart disease.

For these reasons, everybody should be strongly advised to cut down or, if possible, stop their smoking. People who rely a great deal on smoking for comfort may find it difficult to stop, and we must never force them against their will. We must avoid being cruel in our attempts to improve their health. Interestingly, many dementia sufferers forget about a lifelong smoking habit and give it up quite easily.

5 Constipation and diarrhoea

Many older people have problems with constipation. Lifelong diets that are low in roughage (fibre) may contribute to this, but many people also find that their bowels just do not move as readily as they used to, or that the body's message that they need the toilet does not come so clearly. Add to this the facts that they:

- may not exercise enough
- may not drink enough fluids in over-heated buildings
- may not be taking enough roughage
- may be taking medicines that tend to cause constipation as an unwanted effect
- may forget whether they have been to the toilet

and we have a recipe for major problems.

Mr Ho, over a period of a few days, was found wandering around the Home during the night and seemed to be more agitated and anxious during the day. Cathy, his care worker, was very concerned and reported that he was showing signs of disturbed behaviour. She had found him spreading faeces around the toilet. The doctor had been called and prescribed a tranquilliser, but things became no better as Mr Ho became more confused and was not going to the toilet. The doctor was asked to re-visit and on this occasion diagnosed that Mr Ho had constipation.

Constipation in dementia is one of the chief causes of distress, restlessness, sleeplessness, lethargy, pain and physical decline. Mr Ho might have had a blockage high up in his bowel, in which normal control of the bowel is lost and results in diarrhoea. Giving him a 'binding' medicine could result in making his condition worse. Of course, diarrhoea can also be caused by an infection, by diverticulitis, or even by too much treatment for constipation(!), so finding out what is going on will require special medical expertise and may need special tests, such as an x-ray of the patient's abdomen.

In Mr Ho's situation, problems arose because he made attempts to deal with his constipation. He tried to use his fingers to help empty his bowel, and ended up smearing faeces around the toilet. This looks like so-called 'disturbed behaviour' and might even tempt staff to give a tranquilliser.

But Mr Ho needed more understanding care: the change in his bowel habit was reported to the doctor, who was asked to investigate.

6 Incontinence

Incontinence problems of various kinds are very common among otherwise healthy older people, and there are many causes. Simple causes such as urinary infections, too-high doses of diuretic medicines ('water pills'), or doses given at the wrong time of day, constipation affecting the mechanics of urination, and prostate problems in men, are all common but can be corrected and are worth getting quickly sorted out. In addition, we now know a lot about how the bladder works, and about changes that often occur in older people, making it smaller, weaker or more irritable.

As with constipation, older people may find that the body's messages that they need to pass water may not be as clear as they were. In dementia this tendency is greater, and eventually the control of the brain over the bladder is lost completely, so that people with severe dementia become regularly incontinent. In late stages the same happens to control over the bowels, and faecal incontinence is common in severe dementia. However, in milder dementia, we do not expect incontinence and certainly not incontinence of faeces.

Any new incontinence needs medical assessment; it should never be assumed that it is simply due to the dementia.

Some incontinent 'behaviour' is not actually due to a medical problem. A person who is near to the stage where they might develop incontinence at night may have the problem because they are drinking large quantities of tea before bed time or having alcohol in the evening. The problem is solved by making sure that they drink plenty of fluids during the day but less in the evening. Other people may be 'incontinent' simply because they do not remember where the toilet is, or cannot work their buttons, or cannot get themselves on and off the toilet. Once you know the cause, you can take steps to solve the problem: for instance, a clearer sign on the toilet door, different trouser fastenings or handrails.

Other people may have a problem of judgement: they lose their sense of social right and wrong, and urinate in the middle of the sitting room, not seeming to care that they are offending their neighbours. These people need particular attention. Sometimes an adult conversation, in which you make it clear that such behaviour offends people, can work. More often you need to understand why they are behaving in this way. You can do this by trying to find out what seems to lead to such behaviour and what happens afterwards. It may be that something makes them very angry: perhaps you can find ways to help them get over their anger or even to prevent such a situation. In some instances it may be that they want more of your attention: you might be able to give them special attention at certain times and to make no fuss about the offensive behaviour. With some people you have to encourage them very regularly, and privately suggest the need to go to the toilet to prevent the problem arising.

7 Eyesight and hearing problems

Dementia is not a cause of blindness or deafness, though it does cause the sufferers to gradually understand less and less of what they see or hear. But eyesight and hearing problems are common in older people. People with dementia need all their faculties if they are to retain any independence, so they need special attention to these health problems. The difficulty is that they may not complain, they may forget that they need glasses or a hearing aid, or they may refuse to wear them, thinking that they do not need them. We must not be tempted into thinking that all their problems are due to the dementia. The effects of getting a new pair of glasses or of using a hearing aid or a special communicator can be quite miraculous.

8 Strokes, fits, falls and turns

In all types of dementia, but especially in dementia due to vascular disease and dementia related to Parkinson's disease, mobility problems are common. This is especially so in the later stages of the illness. As with bowel and bladder problems, though, mobility problems arising early in dementia should always be carefully assessed by a doctor.

In multi-infarct and other vascular dementias, strokes may occur. Indeed, they can also occur during the course of Alzheimer-type dementia, because the blood vessels are damaged in that condition as well. Strokes can take many different forms, not only paralysis or speech difficulties. Some merely cause a period of confusion lasting anything from a few minutes to days or a few weeks. Some cause a short period of dizziness. Some are so 'silent' that we notice nothing except the continuing gradual decline caused by the dementia.

Full-scale epileptic fits and lesser fits where the individual has a short period of unconsciousness, or a brief fit of shaking, are very common in the later stages of dementia. Inform the doctor if they occur more than once.

Many other less clear-cut 'turns' occur during the course of dementia, and may lead to unsteadiness or falls. As with the other problems we have been discussing, these can be due to any of a number of causes, including unwanted effects of medication, and many common illnesses such as Parkinson's disease, infections, constipation, heart irregularities and other problems.

Falls may be due to many different causes, including:

- poor coordination;
- poor eyesight;
- badly fitting shoes;
- the wrong walking aid;
- problems with their feet;
- interference by other people;
- badly placed furniture.

Whatever the cause, we should never assume that it is 'just the dementia'. Turns and falls need medical investigation by the doctor.

9 Medication for medical conditions

People with dementia often also have other medical conditions. Some of them will understand this and know how and when to take their medication, but more will need guidance. They will need an arrangement whereby you at least remind them of medication times, or you may have to dispense the drug to them.

Some people may have difficulty swallowing tablets or dislike the taste of particular medicines, or they may refuse to take any medication at all. If you disguise the medication – perhaps crushing a tablet into cornflakes and milk – make sure that this does not limit the effect of the medication.

For example, some tablets have special coatings that are designed to allow a slow-release effect of the drug into the body. Find out from the doctor, pharmacist or a senior member of staff why the medication has been prescribed and the possible unwanted (side) effects.

You should remember that, though you may be giving medication because you are acting in the person's best interests, if this is done without that individual's consent it could be a criminal offence. In Chapter 8 we deal with legal aspects in more detail.

The times when medication is taken can be very important. For example, should it be taken before, with or after meals? And does an instruction 'three times a day' mean during the day time or spread through 24 hours (every eight hours – 8 am, 4 pm and midnight)? Not following instructions carefully can add to medical problems instead of making them better.

As well as being on the lookout for any unwanted effects, check that the beneficial effects are there – that the drug is working properly. The individuals may well be unlikely to judge this themselves. It is also important to remind the doctor if someone has been getting repeat prescriptions of a medicine for some time. Is the medicine still needed? If so, is the dose still the right one?

10 Medication for disturbed behaviour

Better education about dementia and better support for staff in day care centres and residential homes, as well as better education of doctors, should be gradually reducing the use of drugs to deal with problem behaviour. In the past there was a tendency to over-prescribe sleeping tablets, rather than asking whether there was a real problem or looking into the causes of the sleeplessness. Behaviour problems by day are often due to medical conditions, or to distress which can be dealt with more imaginatively, or to lack of or over-stimulation which can be cured. Nevertheless, there are some times when drug treatments are both necessary and appropriate.

Few of the tranquilliser and anti-depressant medicines that are used in this way are free from unwanted effects. Some people, and especially people with dementia, are extremely sensitive to some tranquilliser drugs and 'normal' doses may be bad for them. For these reasons you should never allow a situation where a doctor prescribes a drug for disturbed behaviour without proper medical and psychological assessment, and without seeing whether other measures might be more effective. You should never start a new drug of this type unless you know that you can quickly get the doctor back if it does not work or has unwanted effects. You should always ask for information on the effects (good *and* unwanted) to be available for all staff. And you should ask for regular reviews of the need for such drugs and for reviews of the dosage.

Detecting medical problems in dementia, bringing them to the doctors' attention and helping in their management are important tasks for all the staff of care homes and day care centres. The patient will not necessarily be able to complain properly, or to help easily in investigation or treatment. There may be limits to how far you go with treatment. Doctors may seem reluctant to get too involved. But you must never assume that all a person's problems are due to dementia. People with dementia deserve good medical and nursing help just as much as anybody. If they get second best, they suffer unnecessary distress, and our ability to help them live comfortably and happily is severely diminished.

KEY POINTS

- When someone with dementia rapidly becomes confused, this may be a delirium.
- Arrange regular six-monthly checks of the person's health.
- Ensure a good balanced diet and regular activity.
- Not all incontinence problems are due to dementia.
- Staff should know of the unwanted effects of prescribed 'cocktails' of drugs.
- Staff should always bring to the doctor's attention any sudden changes in the health of a resident with dementia.

TRAINING EXERCISES

1   Over the last week an individual has been refusing to eat, despite being given
    a lot of encouragement. She does drink enough. What might be possible
    explanations?

2   An individual has recently become incontinent and is plainly distressed by it. The
    incontinence adviser suggests using pads, but this has increased the distress
    of the person, who sees them as nappies. What else might be considered?

8 Legal Issues

This chapter looks at how the law applies to people with dementia in residential and day care and discusses when it might be helpful to use it.

MAKING DECISIONS

Dementia affects the person's ability to understand, concentrate and remember, as well as interfering with the ability to carry out daily living tasks. It is not surprising, then, that it also affects the person's ability to make choices and decisions. This can range from the difficulties deciding what to eat for lunch or working out when is an appropriate time to go for a walk to dealing with finances or giving consent for medical treatment.

Many people with dementia can state their preferences. For others you can work out what their preference might be because you know what kind of person they were before the illness and how they might have decided. This is fine for most kinds of decisions. When there is a risk, though, of the person with dementia hurting themselves or others, or there is a risk of financial loss, and you are worried that they may be unable to understand the consequences of any decisions they make, you have to look at what guidance the law offers.

THE LAW AND MENTAL HEALTH

First let us deal with the risk of someone hurting themselves.

Mrs Amble keeps trying to leave the building. You know she cannot find her way back and you are fearful of her falling or getting run over. You want to safeguard her by locking the door. You are caught between your duty to protect her and her right to decide for herself.

You have a 'duty of care' which means in this context that her welfare should be your first concern. She also has rights under Common Law to decide for herself up to a point. You have to draw a fine balance between restraint and allowing people to decide for themselves as far as possible. Restraint must not be cruel and must never be used without first carefully considering the alternatives.

It is all too easy to assume that the resident with dementia is simply unable to make all important decisions and to treat them like children. Some families and care staff do this, thinking it more kindly to decide for Mrs Amble because she is unable to explain why she wants to leave and gives no indication that she understands the risks involved. Many people with dementia do not have Mrs Amble's determination and seem quite happy to let you decide on their behalf. They would not object, as she does, to having the door locked. But this lack of objection does not make it right for staff to take decisions for people in their care.

The reason for locking her in would be to protect her from risk, but the risk must be clear, substantial and proven, and your action would need to be the minimum necessary. Good practice demands that no individual makes a decision to restrain anyone in any way. These decisions should always be made jointly, involving the individual, the family and the staff. The decision should be thoroughly recorded, and should include any dissenting views and a record of how the decision was reached, what alternatives were considered and evidence that the restraint used is the minimum necessary.

This book has emphasised the principle of assisting people with dementia to have as much independence as possible. We have stressed the need to enhance self-esteem and dignity whenever possible. Taking decisions for people does not usually enhance their confidence even though it may be well meaning. Instead we should try at all times to keep people in charge of their lives for as long as they are able, even if it means taking some risks. Instead of choosing for the person, we need to help them see – in the simplest way possible – what their choices are.

Consent

'Consent' is a technical term. In general, to give proper legal consent, a person has to be:

- mentally capable of understanding an explanation, in broad terms and simple language, of the basic information relevant to the decision to be made;
- able to make a choice;
- able to communicate in some way;
- not under any undue pressure.

It is important to look at the particular decision in question and at the individual's capacity to make that decision in the context of their own personal circumstances. For some decisions, there are specific legal tests of capacity defined in the law; for example, the test of capacity to manage financial affairs is different from the test of capacity to consent to medical treatment.

Clearly, many people with dementia are unable to make particular decisions. Once again you are caught between the duty to care for someone and their right to decide. Legally, if you take away their right to decide you must have the sanction of the law.

Most of the time, responsible decisions relating to the day-to-day care of the person can be made in consultation with the relatives and by knowing the person well. Sometimes you will find that having the information and the options explained simply will enable the person with dementia to decide. It is often worth considering using an advocate. This is someone who is brought into discussions to represent the wishes of the individual, especially someone without actively involved relatives. This can be on the basis of a long-term relationship with the individual or for the specific episode. Advocacy schemes are not very well developed but you might well find a relative, friend, solicitor or community nurse willing to take on this role.

You may feel that Mrs Amble is no longer able to make the decision for herself about when she goes out of the Home. This is not a viewpoint to be taken lightly. In Mrs Amble's case there is no family to talk it over with, but this should ideally be the first step if you ever take such a view of a resident. There are then a whole set of steps that can be taken before any form of restraint is considered:

1 Staff should get together with the family (if there is one) and the individual if possible, to discuss the reasons why Mrs Amble keeps wanting to go out. Perhaps there are not enough activities and she is bored, perhaps something is distressing her, perhaps it is the side effects of drugs or she is disorientated, perhaps she is angry, and so on. There are positive things that can be done about all of these.

2 If her behaviour is new the doctor should be called to check if there is a medical cause or treatment. The doctor might refer her for a specialist assessment.

3 The circumstances of the placement should be considered. Is she in the right room and does she have her own possessions around her? Does she get on with her room mate, is she in the right Home, does she ever have visitors? Is everything possible done to ensure that she can find her way around the Home?

4 Is there a problem in the staff attitudes to Mrs Amble which is making her feel unwelcome or unwanted?

Guardianship

You may occasionally be asked to look after a resident who is under Guardianship. It might have been the way someone like Mrs Amble arrived in your Home if she had been felt to be at great risk to herself at home and yet refused the alternatives.

A Guardian may be appointed for a person who is suffering from mental disorder, if it is necessary for the welfare of that person or for the protection of others. A Guardian has power to require the person under Guardianship to follow certain courses of action (see below). An application for reception into Guardianship may be made under the Mental Health Act 1983 in England and Wales (or the Mental Health Act Scotland 1984, or Mental Health (Northern Ireland) Order 1986). The application is made to the local social services authority, and must be supported by two doctors and an Approved Social Worker (Mental Welfare Officer or

Mental Health Officer), who must agree that the person is suffering from a mental disorder of a nature or degree that warrants reception into Guardianship. The application can be made by an Approved Social Worker or by the person's nearest relative. The Approved Social Worker must report on the individual's welfare and indicate how it will be helped by appointing a Guardian. A Guardian will be appointed if the local authority is satisfied that this is necessary for the person's welfare or for the protection of others. The only powers available to a Guardian are to require the person:

- to live at a specified address (eg a residential home);
- to attend somewhere such as a day centre or clinic for the purposes of receiving medical treatment, occupation, education or training;
- to allow access to named people such as a doctor or social worker.

The Guardian can be an individual (such as a relative) but it is more usually the local authority. The Guardian cannot consent to medical or psychiatric treatment or make financial decisions for their 'ward'.

You should not be frightened of Guardianship. The need for Guardianship is regularly reviewed by the local social services authority, who are usually the Guardians, and by the Mental Health Act Commission (Mental Welfare Commission in Scotland, and, in some circumstances, the Mental Health Review Tribunal in Northern Ireland). So you can be sure that proper safeguards are in place.

Other Sections

What about other sections of the Mental Health or equivalent legislation? These are mostly concerned with the harm or injury someone is doing to themselves or others and where compulsory removal to and detention in a hospital is necessary. You might have a resident who was hitting other residents with a Zimmer frame in unprovoked attacks. It is likely that you would speedily involve the GP, who would in turn involve a psychiatrist. In these circumstances you do not need to be aware of the specifics of the legislation.

Consent to treatment

If a resident is competent, the right exists under Common Law for them to consent to or refuse medical treatment. You need to be sure they have all the information about the benefits and risks of the proposed treatments and possible alternatives to it, that they are able to weigh these up and that they understand what you are explaining to them. A person's capacity to consent may fluctuate, so it is important to choose the best time to talk to them when they are most lucid.

If the resident is not capable of giving their own consent, there is no power in law for someone to give consent for them. However, the courts have accepted that treatment can be carried out by a doctor if it is in the best interests of the patient. Where a treatment is irreversible, application must be made to the courts before action can be taken.

If we find illnesses that are serious, complicated or difficult to treat we should not necessarily rush in to demanding treatment in every case except in an emergency. There is a balance to be drawn.

Suppose that Mr Ho was found to have cancer of the bowel. In considering whether he needs complicated or perhaps painful treatment, we need to bear in mind his overall emotional and physical well-being and understanding. Treatment might cause further confusion or worsen the condition in other ways. Mr Ho may be unlikely to be seen as legally able to give consent to surgery, so a decision may have to be made for him.

Every situation is different and the decision must rest with the doctor proposing the treatment. It is the effects on the individual resident and their family that are the main considerations. It might be right to treat Mr Ho's cancer and give him the possibility of a more comfortable few years. It might be kinder to let the illness run its course whilst keeping him as comfortable as possible. Mr Ho is lucky to have an involved family who have his best interests at heart, but suppose it was Mrs Amble who had cancer of the lung. Who should be involved in making the best possible decision for her? Once again, an advocate might be helpful to ensure that her perspective has been thoroughly considered.

Ultimately, it is the doctor proposing the treatment who must decide what is in the person's best interests, taking into account the patient's views (past and present) and the views of relatives, carers and other medical staff.

You may occasionally come across a resident who has made a 'living will' (also called an 'advance directive'). Although this has no formal legal status it is a record made by someone when in their right mind about what they want to happen in the event of life-threatening illness or injury when they may be unable to be consulted. It can be a great help in making decisions because at least this document can be considered with all the other points of view. In a recent case, a patient's right to give or refuse consent to future medical treatment by way of an advance directive was recognised by the High Court.

However, we must not assume that people with dementia are less likely to want treatment than the rest of us. Many younger people, imagining the deterioration and distress caused by dementia, think that people with the illness would want to be allowed to die. The reality is that, although dementia is distressing for relatives and other carers, it is not always distressing for the person. Another fact to bear in mind is that people with dementia are often able to talk about death if they feel comfortable and will express views about their own death.

This whole issue is very difficult because a balance has to be made between the duty to care (that is, not to neglect the individual) and the duty not to make them undergo distressing or painful treatments without very good reason. Legally the balance has always been towards the duty to care, so staff are in general protected if they take action in good faith to help mentally incompetent people in their charge to avoid distress, suffering or injury, even if this means actions that in other circumstances would be seen as interference.

Section 47 of the National Assistance Act

You may very occasionally be asked to provide accommodation under section 47 of the National Assistance Act 1948. This Act provides for the compulsory removal of older people from their home for a short period if they are at risk. They must be 'suffering from grave chronic disease or, being aged, infirm or physically incapacitated, are living in insanitary conditions and are unable to devote to themselves, and are not receiving from other persons, proper care and attention'.

You should be very wary of this if the person has dementia. People with dementia are more properly dealt with under the mental health legislation.

So far we have looked at the way the law protects people's safety. We will now move on to consider the use of the law in relation to people's money.

Protecting the assets of your residents

Staff may find that they become involved in helping residents to spend their money. Under the Residential Care Homes Regulations, the Home must provide a place where money and valuables can be deposited for safe-keeping, and must keep a record of all money deposited or that they have received on the resident's behalf. In default of detailed guidance, the Social Services Inspectorate have advised the use of *Other People's Money*, published by Age Concern England (see p 136), which gives guidance on the responsibilities of formal carers in the National Health Service.

Agents and Appointees

The simplest way to help a person with dementia who still has the ability to manage their money is to become their *Agent*. This allows someone to act on the individual's behalf, for the purpose of collecting state benefits. Do note, however, that the person must still sign for the benefit and be legally competent to agree to the arrangement. Although there is no check made on such arrangements, it is essential to keep careful records.

In many cases the easiest solution would be for the Home's manager to act as Agent. However, *Home Life*, the code of practice for residential care, advises that proprietors or managers should not take on this role unless it has proved impossible to find an alternative.

If a person with dementia is not capable of managing their own financial affairs and needs help with state benefits, it is possible to apply to be an *Appointee*. Appointed by the Secretary of State, the Appointee (who is probably a relative) will claim, receive and deal with payments from the Benefits Agency on behalf of, and for the benefit of, the individual. Application is made in writing to the Benefits Agency and they have to satisfy themselves that the individual is unable to manage their financial affairs. This is usually carried out by means of a letter from a doctor and sometimes a visit to meet you and the individual. Again, staff of care homes should not become involved in taking on this role because of the risk of abuse and conflict of interest. If a member of staff becomes an Appointee, the Benefits Agency has a duty to inform the Registering Authority.

Appointeeship requires there to be a decision about the person's legal competence. Usually the GP can decide on this, based on whether the person has any understanding, their level of confusion and their abilities and skills to deal with their own affairs. This will, of course, depend on how complicated (or otherwise) their particular affairs are. If you suspect that an Appointee is failing in their duty to the individual, you should inform the Home's manager. If the matter is not resolved satisfactorily, it can be raised with the Benefits Agency.

Powers of Attorney and Enduring Powers of Attorney

A Power of Attorney allows a person to give someone the power to act on their behalf, either in general financial affairs or in a specific financial transaction. It can be given only by a person who is 'competent' (the relevant test of capacity to make an Enduring Power of Attorney is defined in case law). In England and Wales (but not in Scotland), an ordinary Power of Attorney becomes invalid when the person becomes incompetent. An Enduring Power of Attorney, however, remains valid so long as it is registered with the Court of Protection (part of the Supreme Court that deals with the financial affairs of mentally incapacitated people). If an Attorney under an Enduring Power, which has been registered, appears to be abusing that power, complaints can be made to the Court of Protection, who should investigate.

You may come across these Powers of Attorney in two ways. First, you will have residents who have given their relatives Power of Attorney or Enduring Power of Attorney. If the resident has become ill with dementia since the Powers were given, you need to be alert to the fact that the first will be invalid. If, for example, Mrs Begum had given Power of Attorney rather than Enduring Power of Attorney to her children before going into the Home, it would be invalid once she became unable to manage her own affairs by reason of her dementia. The second way you may come across it is if a resident or client asks you to act as their attorney. You should not agree to this, because it could be misinterpreted. It would certainly be invalid unless they were legally competent.

The Court of Protection, Curator Bonis and Office of Care and Protection

The Court of Protection in England and Wales, Curators Bonis in Scotland and the Office of Care and Protection in Northern Ireland all have wide powers to manage the financial affairs of people who, because of mental disorder, are unable to manage their own affairs and are unable to grant a Power of Attorney. An application should be made if a mentally incapacitated individual's affairs are too complicated to be dealt with by an Appointee and no previous arrangements have been made (eg to make an Enduring Power of Attorney). The Court will need to be satisfied, after considering medical evidence, that the individual concerned is incapable of managing their own affairs because of mental disorder.

The Court of Protection and the Office of Care and Protection both can appoint a *Receiver*, who will usually be a relative but may be a professional such as a solicitor or accountant. In Scotland a Court of Session or local Sheriff Court can appoint a financial manager, called a *Curator Bonis*. These actions are usually relevant only if the person has savings of more than around £5,000 (or at least £10,000 in Scotland), or if their affairs are at all complicated. For someone with only limited assets, the Court in England and Wales may make a Short Procedure Order, giving directions as to how the individual's affairs should be organised. In Scotland, in certain circumstances the local authority may pay for a Curator Bonis.

Wills

In order to draw up a valid Will a person must have 'testamentary capacity': that is, they must have an understanding of the extent of their assets and of what the Will is for, and an awareness of their obligations towards relatives and friends who might expect to inherit under the Will (even if they do not wish to act on them). In addition, they must not be too easily swayed by undue pressure about the terms of the Will. It would be advisable for an individual to seek legal advice in drawing up a Will, and a medical opinion may be necessary to make sure they have testamentary capacity. It is possible for the Court of Protection to make a 'statutory Will' for people who no longer have testamentary capacity, for whom a Receiver has been appointed or who have a registered Enduring Power of Attorney. It is very unwise for staff to allow themselves to be named as beneficiaries. If it is suggested that you may be named in a Will, you should discuss this fully with your manager.

Related to this is the thorny question of whether staff should accept gifts from residents. It could be very hurtful for Mrs Begum, for example, if staff she regards as friends refuse her gifts. Staff should be encouraged to accept small gifts gracefully but should let their manager know if bigger ones are offered so that this can be discussed with the relatives.

COMPLAINTS

Complaints procedures relate to both safety matters and financial matters, so they are considered last here. Under the National Health Service and Community Care Act, each authority must have a complaints procedure. If you are running a voluntary or private home you will be asked to set one up.

A complaints procedure can be very useful in getting feedback from residents or clients and relatives but this is much more difficult with people who have dementia. Mrs Amble may well have a lot of complaints, Mr Ho and Mrs Begum none. This does not mean that they or their relatives might not want to make some comments on the running of the Home.

It is important that residents or clients and their families understand how complaints are dealt with and that they are welcomed as a way of improving the service that you offer. However, there will be occasions when people with dementia make false accusations. You will remember that Mrs Begum made accusations when she was beginning to lose her memory and was very distressed about it. Staff should be encouraged to talk about such accusations and to see the reasons for them.

It is very important to have sound financial procedures and records so that there is no chance that accusations about money cannot be defended with written documentation. If, for example, Mrs Begum had asked for some items of shopping, you should ensure that another staff member is present both when the request is made and when giving her the items, the receipts and her change.

If accusations persist, even if you believe them to be false, then outside help is required – if for no other reason than to protect your good name.

A social worker, solicitor or doctor may be the right person, depending on the particular situation. It is bad practice to have a resident continually complaining or making accusations against the staff, who seem to be ignoring her or, worse still, laughing off the accusations.

You may occasionally come across a situation in which it may seem that relatives or others are not acting in the best interests of the individual; for example, in handling their financial affairs. If you suspect abuse or exploitation, it is important to raise these concerns with your manager, and possibly with a social worker, so that it can be reported to the relevant authorities and action can be taken to safeguard the individual's interests.

A NOTE TO MANAGERS

This chapter has explained the law but it has not gone into any great detail because you are unlikely to need this. If you are concerned about the meaning or implications of parts of the Mental Health legislation, you might like to invite the Approved Social Worker (Mental Welfare Officer) from your local social services/social work office to do a training session for you and your staff.

KEY POINTS

- There are laws that protect people with dementia.
- There are a great many steps to take before considering any form of restraint.
- To give legal 'consent' or to make a will, a person must understand what the particular decision is all about, be able to communicate their decision and not be under any pressure.
- To make important decisions for someone else about their finances or medical treatment, you must have sanction of the law.
- It is important to have a proper complaints procedure in place to protect both residents and staff.

TRAINING EXERCISE

Think about one of your troubling residents or day care clients with dementia and list what you imagine to be the solution as seen by all the different parties involved: the GP, the relatives, the different staff who work with him or her, etc. You might find it interesting to write down the justification different people give for their ideas.

9 A Staff Survival Kit

This chapter is about you and coping with the extra demands of caring for people with dementia.

TYPICAL RESPONSES

At times coping will seem daunting to staff teams, especially as there will be occasions when things go unexpectedly wrong, despite all good caring practice and good intentions.

When something goes wrong, a typical response of many teams is:

- to blame a colleague;
- to feel that they do not have the necessary skills or knowledge;
- to complain that caring for people with dementia is too demanding and unrewarding, and not the caring they want to do;
- to blame the management for expecting them to cope without enough staff;
- to confirm their view that people with dementia are over-dependent and unpredictable.

Perhaps these views have been voiced in your team? If so, they may reflect the fact that you are often so caught up in the dilemmas, pressures and responsibilities of the job that you forget the importance of valuing each other's personal abilities as team members.

All too often staff set themselves the unrealistic objective of being all things to all people and forget that personalities can sometimes clash. It is no admission of failure to realise that you can find it hard to relate to one resident or day care client whilst others present no difficulty. Teams need to spend time thinking about the hobbies, interests and life experiences of individual care staff that could be used to help them respond positively to a 'difficult' person.

A positive team of permanent staff can:

- create an atmosphere that encourages staff to develop and improve skills;
- enable staff to develop a deeper knowledge of the residents or clients in their unit, making it easier to identify changes in behaviour;
- use their knowledge of residents or clients to predict the resources required to meet their changing needs;
- achieve better care by working together.

Like family carers at home, staff carers need respite. No matter how good we are at our job, the task of caring for dementia sufferers is stressful. If staff are finding that an individual is causing them great stress by his or her degree of dependence, or behaviour or distress, it is not unreasonable to ask for some respite from the task of caring. This might in some cases mean bringing in extra outside help. It might mean arranging special outings with relatives or a paid helper. In a Home it might mean arranging for the person to have day care in a day centre or day hospital. And it might mean respite care in hospital, perhaps even on a regular basis. The combination of the best possible management in the Home or day centre, good support for staff, outside advice and respite if necessary should result in continuity of care. Few residents in a good Home in good communication with other services need to be shifted to other Homes or hospitals even when they are in the advanced stages of dementia.

COMMUNICATION

Team members often communicate about the wrong things! We are so busy discussing the day-to-day tasks that we forget to stop and think about how we are functioning as a team.

Working with people with dementia can be very stressful. There may be times when all our efforts to respond in a caring and sensitive way get no reaction from the individual or, alternatively, get an explosion of emotional feeling. On such occasions it is important for the team to give support to the staff member involved. This support does not just happen – everyone in the team must have a clear sense of their purpose and agree how they will put this into practice.

A NOTE FOR MANAGERS

Managing teams of staff and self-management are extremely difficult tasks. Every individual person is a mixture of feelings, attitudes, thoughts, prejudices, skills, strengths and weaknesses, which can be difficult enough to cope with. But put a group of individuals together, be they a staff team or people with dementia, the problem is even bigger.

The whole caring profession is experiencing a time of change, bringing with it new traumas and challenges. Never has the work of managing people been so vital within the profession. Managers often find themselves in this role with little or no management training. You may have knowledge and skills in client care, have hopes and aspirations of the care you want to provide, but there is no time to consider this important role and how best to function.

Begin now by asking two basic questions:

1 What is my organisation trying to achieve?
2 How do I think I should provide care to people with dementia?

It is important to stand back and look at the context in which we work before grappling with the 'nitty gritty' of what goes on. Thinking about both questions is important because you need to be sure about the purpose of your work. Is it about rehabilitation, or is it about helping people with dementia to lead as normal a life as possible?

TRAINING

Training is not the answer for all ills!

Providing a staff development and training programme shows that managers recognise the demands made on staff. Such a programme should be seen as a long-term continuing investment in staff morale, knowledge, skills and awareness.

All too often, staff training has been provided only when something has gone wrong, and a specially arranged session has been organised. But training is not a cure for the ills of poorly thought out procedures, inappropriate routines or a lack of philosophy of care which are often the hallmarks of poor management. A good Home or day care centre has a regular training programme for staff, and also provides education and support for relatives and other carers.

Valuing staff and each other

Staff need to feel valued, skilled and recognised for the good care they provide. Training opportunities can encourage team members to share new learning and explore with colleagues some of the dilemmas and problems they encounter.

Colleagues can:

- help each other;
- gain support from each other;
- try out new ideas;
- evaluate each other's work.

The following are some suggestions for achieving good teamwork and practical support for each other.

Use 'hand-over' meetings between shifts to evaluate and review work

Too often these meetings are predictable, superficial comments about residents or clients. They can be more productive when they are also used to evaluate care plans and check whether goals are being achieved or whether changes are required.

Arrange regular supervision on a one-to-one basis

Supervision should be an interactive process that is a firm part of a relationship in which all parties contract to undertake work on clearly agreed objectives. Working together on a one-to-one basis encourages discussion of new or extra training needs.

Organise small team forums

Small groups of four or five people can meet to discuss important issues. The manager need not lead this forum but team members could each take responsibility for a particular topic.

Have regular staff meetings to further team development

Meetings should not be occasions to be endured where only one or a few people contribute and where some managers use the opportunity to lay down the rules. The quality of meetings can usually be judged by the way people either look forward to or dread the normal weekly or monthly get-together. How do you feel about meetings in your Home or day care centre? Could you contribute more, or better, perhaps?

Plan for special interest meetings

Inviting colleagues from other fields can stimulate and improve the quality of collaborative work as ideas and experiences are shared. Community nurses, occupational therapists, home care assistants, carers of people with dementia living at home can all add to the bank of knowledge and skills.

Use local resources

Local colleges and libraries can supply books and articles on subjects related to dementia. These can be reviewed and discussed by staff, so keeping in touch with current thinking and practice.

Valuable contributions can also be made by people from voluntary groups, carers groups, and friends and relatives of your residents or clients. You can all learn from each other.

THE DEVELOPING TEAM

If a team is to be effective it needs to keep developing itself, and this means individual as well as team development. The various types of supervision should be explored and agreement reached on the ones that suit your particular situation. This will go a long way towards helping everyone to perform at their highest level.

People in the team need to be honest and not feel they are failing if some situations are hard to handle, such as an individual's repetitive behaviour which irritates intensely. Admit it and then the issue can be tackled collectively. In an effective team people can, and do, express themselves openly and honestly. Mistakes and difficult situations are faced and used to learn from.

People who work in care homes or day centres do so for a variety of reasons. Although they may be motivated by a concern for older people, they also have needs and expectations. Being valued and appreciated as a member of staff not only will help that person to feel that what they do is worthwhile but also will help build team morale.

Caring for people with dementia has many 'highs' and 'lows'. Work will not always be a happy, stress-free experience, so managers should consider how they are providing opportunities for learning, developing skills and a greater awareness of needs. A clearly thought out training strategy and staff development policy can be an important part of this work.

KEY POINTS

- Effective teams support, help and value each other's contribution.

- Training is not a cure for all ills, but will help to develop and improve skills.

- Supervision and meetings can be used to encourage individual and team development.

- Staff may need respite from particularly demanding residents with dementia.

TRAINING EXERCISE

Think of a staff team of which you were a member or are a member now. The team might be the regular group of colleagues you are on shift with. Ask yourself: what are the good points of being in this team?

Then think about the question: is there one thing that we could improve upon so as to work more as a team?

Appendix 1

MODEL ANSWERS TO TRAINING EXERCISES

Here are our suggested responses to the exercises, which were aimed at prompting healthy discussion and leading to good care practice.

Chapter 1
Caring for the individual

On admission, it would be important for the person with dementia to know someone already, a familiar face they would recognise. People for whom English is a second (and perhaps forgotten) language need someone there who speaks their first language. This could be a relative who came with them from their own home, a staff member or even another resident who had perhaps lived nearby.

Because unfamiliar surroundings create anxiety for the person with dementia, it would help their orientation if they were shown only the important places first time round (ie toilet, bedroom, dining room). Familiar objects from their own home might help to reassure them. The 'buddy' system of pairing another resident with the newcomer is one way of avoiding some early problems.

Make sure that new residents and day care clients know who you are and where they are and what's happening to them!

Chapter 2
Understanding and care

Although people have labelled both Mr Ho and Mrs Amble as having dementia, you should be sure that they are assessed and diagnosed correctly. Mr Ho, for instance, has multi-infarct dementia but his lethargy might be a result of some medication he is taking that the GP forgot to mention. You would contact the doctor anyway but in Mr Ho's case you might want to talk to him through an interpreter to find out how he is feeling, rather than rely on what the family might tell you.

As our feeling of self-worth is based on how others react to us, it is important to treat each person with respect and dignity which acknowledge that individual's previous lifestyle. Reminiscence and life story books have a part to play here.

Chapter 3
Working with dementia

1   One method of finding out about an individual is to compile a life story book with them and their relatives and friends. This can be a useful cue for staff in discussing with the person their memories of school, work and what it was like to live in the 1930s and 1940s.

2   Sedative syrup should never be given to someone unless it has been prescribed by a doctor. Use of these syrups should be viewed as a last resort and only after other ways of dealing with a situation have not worked. Medication is no substitute for sensitive, insightful and planned responses to a resident's needs.

3   The stages you might have listed for getting up in the morning are:

a   knowing where the different items of clothing are kept

b   deciding what you want to wear

c   remembering to take off the clothes you had on

d   remembering how to put on your underwear

e   putting on the underwear first

f   putting on your shirt/blouse, knowing where to put your arms and remembering to fasten the buttons

g   putting on trousers/skirt and remembering to fasten the waist

h   pulling on socks/tights

i   putting on jersey/pullover/cardigan

j   putting on shoes or slippers – on the correct feet

Getting dressed is more complicated than you thought! So to help a resident with dementia to be independent, the care plan might usefully consider:

■   ways of helping them to know where their different items of clothing are kept;

■   the key worker being with the resident to help them choose the item of clothing they want to wear, and checking how they feel about it;

■   laying out the clothes in the correct sequence;

■   being with the resident and prompting when necessary;

■   praising and complimenting the resident when they complete a task – however small.

You will have residents or day care clients who can manage some aspects of dressing. You might like to reflect on whether helping them has diminished their skills over the months. For example, just because someone puts their clothes on in the wrong sequence does not mean that the staff member should dress them.

Chapter 4
Meaningful routines

1   Although Mrs Amble is now living in a group situation, this is not a common experience for her – or for most of us. It is important for staff to spend time with her, helping her to understand where she is and perhaps encouraging her to make some new friends by introducing her to other residents. More able residents are often happy to be involved in acting as a 'buddy' to help a new resident become accustomed to new routines. It might also help to have some favourite items from her own home – even furniture, if there is space for it.

There is no single solution to problems with residents smoking. Fire regulations often mean that smoke detectors are installed in bedrooms and communal areas, which restricts what can be done. An obvious response would be to have Mrs Amble's cigarettes held by staff so that she would have to ask for (or repeatedly demand) them. (This might create stress for staff, though.) A possible alternative is to encourage Mrs Amble to use the designated smoking area, which most Homes should have. If this area is homely, warm and inviting, Mrs Amble may feel that she likes to be there.

With regard to Mrs Amble walking about at night, it might be that you have to consider the routine of the Home. For instance, if a resident is waking up at night, there may be a number of reasons: noisy domestic staff cleaning communal areas, fear of the dark, being put to bed too early or a lack of stimulating activity through the day. Rather than night staff forcing the resident to go back to bed, if that person is happy being with staff and enjoys a midnight cup of tea then the solution might be to give him or her an opportunity to sit with staff.

2   The kitchen was often the hub of daily activity for many older people and so it is likely that they will remember many of the chores they used to do. Washing and drying dishes, baking or making cups of tea are all activities that can help people with dementia gain some sense of self-esteem. Some individuals may need to be prompted; sometimes they will still do everything wrong or make a mess, even when you have given them guidance and help. Though this can be frustrating for you, it can encourage smiling responses from those involved. Risks are all too evident from hot cooker surfaces, kettles of boiling water and sharp knives. Nevertheless, with careful thought and by working alongside and with the individual, the risk factor can be reduced.

Chapter 5
Dilemmas and challenges

1   Mrs Amble is wanting some sort of sexual relationship. It would be helpful to consider all the people who are involved – the male resident(s), the relatives, other residents and staff – to make sure that no one will be hurt by such a relationship. As long as there does not appear to have been any coercion, there are no grounds to prevent it.

2   Ethical issues might include the consent of the person with dementia (see Chapter 8), whether the person with dementia benefits from it, whether it is used instead of skilled staff or because of poor design, and so on.

Chapter 6
Good design

1   Remember that to many people with dementia the layout of the Home or day centre can be confusing and frightening. It is important to clarify the differences between the doors to their bedroom, a toilet and the dining room. Trying to find their way along a corridor that looks the same as other corridors adds to disorientation, so the addition of some old-fashioned items of furniture, ornaments or pictures can help make a corridor or hall more homely and easier to understand.

People with dementia increasingly depend on visual clues to act as prompts to their orientation and understanding. For example, it will help them to have a coat and hat stand situated in the hall or a piano in the lounge or a welsh dresser in the dining room.

2   Your living room may have something to watch from the window. Pictures and photographs that are familiar, such as local scenes in the 1930s, may help discussion. Some people like to dust and sweep: are dusters and brushes available? Are there plants to be cared for or animals and birds to be attended to? Are there coffee tables so that more able people can serve tea from a trolley and help others? The TV is not an activity unless the programmes stimulate discussion. Background music is rarely helpful unless used in a planned way. Does your sitting room feel like a traditional sitting room so residents know how to behave?

Day centres should have a living room area for the same reasons.

Chapter 7
Health matters

1   Possible explanations for someone refusing to eat include:

■   a physical illness;

■   problems with teeth or dentures;

■   problems with swallowing;

■   gets upset at mealtimes for some reason;

■   dislikes the food;

■   has forgotten how to use a knife and fork;

■   is depressed – possible grief reaction;

■   staff response to refusal may be making things worse.

2   Other possibilities relating to incontinence are:

- Make sure the incontinence is not related to a physical illness.
- Has the individual moved rooms/units and cannot find the toilet?
- Has the individual forgotten how to use the WC (he may have used a bucket in the past)?
- Is the individual drinking too much?

Chapter 8
Legal issues

This exercise will have illustrated how very differently people see the issue of making decisions for people with dementia. There will probably be staff who take a very protective line and others who take a view that people with dementia are adults and should decide for themselves. General practitioners and relatives tend to take a very protective line.

We suggest that you talk with your local Approved Social Worker (Mental Health Officer) or Registration Officer and discuss further some of the aspects we mention in the chapter. You need to be clear about what your role is when people with dementia are showing signs of not being able to manage their affairs.

Chapter 9
A staff survival kit

Working with people who have dementia is stressful. Staff need to feel valued and supported, and to have opportunities to develop their skills and knowledge.

Arranging attendance at training sessions is one way of building a team. We strongly suggest that it is more important to adopt a rigorous approach to regular supervision with individual staff and plan frequent low-cost in-unit training opportunities by use of video, journal articles and case discussion. These can be included as part of a regular team meeting and be prompts for discussion.

Appendix 2

EXTENDED CRICHTON BEHAVIOUR RATING SCALE

MEMORY

Complete	0
Occasionally forgetful	1
Short-term loss	2
Short- and long-term loss	3

ORIENTATION

Complete	0
Orientated in ward, identifies people correctly	1
Misidentifies but can find way out	2
Cannot find way to bed or toilet without assistance	3
Completely lost	4

COMMUNICATION

Always clear, retains information	0
Can indicate needs, understands simple verbal directions, can deal with simple information	1
Cannot understand simple verbal information **or** cannot indicate needs	2
Cannot understand simple verbal information and cannot indicate needs, retains some expressive ability	3
No effective contact	4

CO-OPERATION

Actively co-operative	0
Passively co-operative **or** occasionally unco-operative	1
Requires frequent encouragement or persuasion	2
Rejects assistance, shows independent ill-directed activity	3
Completely resistive or withdrawn	4

RESTLESSNESS

None	0
Intermittent	1
Persistent by day **or** night	2
Persistent by day **and** night	3
Constant	4

AGGRESSIVE BEHAVIOUR

None (may appropriately express anger on occasion)	0
Occasional verbal aggression only	1
Frequent verbal aggression only	2
Verbal aggression and occasional physical aggression	3
Frequent verbal and frequent physical aggression	4

DEMANDING/DISRUPTIVE BEHAVIOUR

None (may make appropriate requests)	0
Occasionally makes repeated requests or repeated questioning	1
Occasionally quite demanding, noisy or disruptive but easily settles	2
Frequently quite demanding/ noisy/ disruptive but easily settles	3
Frequently very demanding/ noisy/disruptive, difficult to settle	4

MOBILITY

Fully ambulant including stairs	0
Usually independent	1
Walks with supervision	2
Walks with aids or under careful supervision	3
Bedfast or chairfast	4

DRESSING

Correct	0
Imperfect but adequate	1
Adequate with minimum supervision	2
Inadequate unless continual supervision	3
Unable to dress **or** to retain clothing	4

FEEDING

Correct unaided at appropriate times	0
Adequate with minimum of supervision	1
Inadequate unless continually supervised	2
Requires feeding	3

BATHING

Washes and bathes without assistance	0
Minimal supervision with bathing	1
Close supervision with bathing	2
Inadequate unless continually supervised	3
Requires washing and bathing	4

CONTINENCE

Full control	0
Occasional accidents	1
Continent by day only if regularly toiletted	2
Urinary incontinence in spite of regular toiletting	3
Regular or frequent double incontinence	4

ENGAGEMENT – ACTIVITIES

Willingly participates in activities and keeps self occupied much of the time	0
Fairly often occupied, participates willingly but may need occasional prompting	1
Occupied only when prompted. Participates only with encouragement	2
Rarely occupied, rarely takes part in activities despite constant encouragement **or** actively refuses to participate	3
Cannot be engaged in any activities, completely passive and withdrawn	4

ENGAGEMENT – SOCIAL

Normal active social contact with others. Initiates conversations. Participates willingly in social activity groups	0
Generally good social contact. Sometimes reluctant to initiate conversation, may need encouragement to talk in groups	1
Spends little time in social contact. Speaks when spoken to. At times can be withdrawn. Occasional interest in conversation. Needs much prompting to join in socially in groups	2
Gives minimum responses only when spoken to. Very little social contact. At times may relate non-verbally (smile, etc.)	3
Completely isolated and withdrawn	4

Useful Addresses

Age Exchange Reminiscence Centre
11 Blackheath Village
London SE3 9LA
Tel: 081-318 9105

Alcohol Concern
32–36 Lamon Street
London SE1 0EE
Tel: 071-928 7377

Alzheimer Scotland – Action on Dementia
8 Hill Street
Edinburgh EH2 3JZ
Tel: 031-225 1453
Helpline: 031-220 6155

Alzheimer's Disease Society
2nd Floor, Gordon House
10 Greencoat Place
London SW1P 1PH
Tel: 071-306 0606

Arthritis and Rheumatism Council for Research
Copeman House
St Mary's Court
St Mary's Gate
Chesterfield S41 7TD
Tel: 0246 558033

Arthritis Care
18 Stephenson Way
London NW1 2HD
Tel: 071-916 1500

British Diabetic Association
10 Queen Anne Street
London W1M 0BD
Tel: 071-323 1531

British Heart Foundation
14 Fitzhardinge Street
London W1H 4DH
Tel: 071-935 0185

British Lung Foundation
8 Peterborough Mews
London SW6 3BL
Tel: 071-371 7704

Cancer Relief Macmillan Fund
Anchor House
15–19 Britten Street
London SW3 3TZ
Tel: 071-351 7811

Carers National Association
20–25 Glasshouse Yard
London EC1A 4JS
Tel: 071-490 8818
Carers Helpline: 071-490 8898
(Mon–Fri, 1–4 pm)

Counsel and Care
Twyman House
16 Bonny Street
London NW1 9PG
Tel: 071-485 1550

Court of Protection
Stewart House
24 Kingsway
London WC2B 6JX
Tel: 071-269 7300

Cruse Bereavement Care
Cruse House
126 Sheen Road
Richmond
Surrey TW9 1UR
Tel: 081-940 4818

Disabled Living Foundation
380–384 Harrow Road
London W9 2HU
Tel: 071-289 6111

Dementia Services Development Centre
University of Stirling
Stirling FK9 4LA
Tel: 0786 467740

Extend (Exercise Training for the Elderly and Disabled)
22 Maltings Drive
Wheathampstead
Herts AL4 8QJ
Tel: 0582 832760

Hospice Information Service
St Christopher's Hospice
51–59 Lawrie Park Road
Sydenham
London SE26 6DZ
Tel: 081-778 9252

Incontinence Information Helpline
c/o Dene Centre
Castle Farm Road
Newcastle-upon-Tyne NE3 1PH
Tel: 091-213 0050
(Mon–Fri, 9 am–6 pm)

MIND (National Association for Mental Health)
Granta House
15–19 Broadway
Stratford
London E15 4BQ
Tel: 081-519 2122

Parkinson's Disease Society
22 Upper Woburn Place
London WC1H 0RA
Tel: 071-383 3513

Royal National Institute for the Blind (RNIB)
224 Great Portland Street
London W1N 6AA
Tel: 071-388 1266

Royal National Institute for Deaf People (RNID)
105 Gower Street
London WC1E 6AH
Tel: 071-387 8033

**SPOD (Association to Aid
the Sexual and Personal
Relationships of People
with a Disability)**
    286 Camden Road
    London N7 0BJ

    Tel: 071-607 8851

**Standing Committee for Ethnic
Minority Senior Citizens**
    5 Westminster Bridge Road
    London SE1 7XW

    Tel: 071-928 0095

Stroke Association
    CHSA House
    123–127 Whitecross Street
    London EC1Y 8JJ

    Tel: 071-490 7999

Terrence Higgins Trust
    52–54 Gray's Inn Road
    London WC1X 8JU

    Tel: 071-831 0330
    Helpline: 071-242 1010 (12–10 pm)

**United Kingdom Home Care
Association (UKHCA)**
    42 Banstead Road
    Carshalton Beaches
    Surrey SM5 3NW

    Tel: 081-770 3658

Further Reading

Activities 2 by Carole Archibald. Dementia Services Development Centre, Stirling, 1993.

Alzheimer's: A care givers' guide and resource book by H Greutzner. John Wiley, New York, 1992.

Common Problems with the Elderly Confused: Aggression by Graham Stokes. Winslow Press, Bicester, Oxon, 1986.

Design in the Context of the Building Regulations by Mary Kelly. Dementia Services Development Centre, Stirling, 1992.

Focus on Restraint. Royal College of Nursing's Forum for the Elderly Mentally Infirm, London, 1987.

Good Care Management by Jenyth Worsley. Age Concern England, London, 1992.

Group Living in Residential Care by Tom Douglas. Tavistock Publications, London, 1988.

Home Life: A code of practice for residential care. Centre for Policy on Ageing, London, 1984.

Life Story Books by Katrina Myers. Dementia Services Development Centre, Stirling, 1991.

Living Well into Old Age: Applying principles of good practice to services for people with dementia. King's Fund Centre, London, 1990.

Living with Dementia: A guide for professionals and carers by John Riordan and Bob Whitmore. Manchester University Press, Manchester, 1990.

The Lost Ones: Using the past to help their present by Faith Gibson. Dementia Services Development Centre, Stirling, 1991.

People with Dementia: The Ferrard approach to care by Faith Gibson. HMSO, London, 1991.

Person to Person: A guide to those with failing mental powers by Tom Kitwood and Kathleen Bredin. Gale House, London, 1992.

Pink Doors and Door Knockers by Nicholas Bell. Dementia Services Development Centre, Stirling, 1992.

A Positive Environment by Ann Netten. Avebury, Aldershot, 1993.

Special Needs Dementia Units: Design, development, operations by Nancy Peppard. Springer, New York, 1991.

Superteams: A blueprint for organizational success by C Hastings, P Bixby and R Chaudry-Lawton. Fontana, London, 1986.

36-Hour Day: A family guide to caring at home for people with Alzheimer's disease and other confusional illnesses by Nancy L Mace and Peter V Rabins. Hodder and Stoughton and Age Concern England, London, 1992.

Understanding Dementia (2nd edition) by Alan Jacques. Churchill Livingstone, Edinburgh, 1992.

Validation: The Feil method by Naomi Feil. Edward Feil, Cleveland, Ohio, 1992.

What If They Hurt Themselves? Counsel and Care, London, 1992.

About Age Concern

Dementia Care: A handbook for residential and day care is one of a wide range of publications produced by Age Concern England, the National Council on Ageing. Age Concern England is actively engaged in training, information provision, fundraising and campaigning for retired people and those who work with them, and also in the provision of products and services, such as insurance, for older people.

A network of over 1,400 local Age Concern groups, with the support of around 250,000 volunteers, aim to improve the quality of life for older people and develop services appropriate to local needs and resources. These include advice and information, day care, visiting services, transport schemes, clubs, and specialist facilities for older people who are physically and mentally frail.

Age Concern England is a registered charity dependent on public support for the continuation and development of its work.

Age Concern England
1268 London Road
London SW16 4ER
Tel: 081-679 8000

Age Concern Cymru
4th Floor
1 Cathedral Road
Cardiff CF1 9SD
Tel: 0222 371566

Age Concern Scotland
54a Fountainbridge
Edinburgh EH3 9PT
Tel: 031-228 5656

Age Concern Northern Ireland
3 Lower Crescent
Belfast BT7 1NR
Tel: 0232 245729

Publications from ◆◆◆ Books

A wide range of titles is published by Age Concern England under the ACE Books imprint.

Health and Care

Taking Good Care: A handbook for care assistants
Jenyth Worsley

Written for professional carers of older people, this book covers such vital issues as the role of the care assistant in a residential home, communication skills, the medical and social problems encountered by carers, the resident's viewpoint and activities and groupwork.

£6.95   0–86242–072–5

Good Care Management: A guide to setting up and managing a residential home
Jenyth Worsley

This companion volume to *Taking Good Care* has been written for care home proprietors and managers, present and prospective. Topics covered include setting up a home, contracts, budgetary planning, staff management and training, the management of care and quality control.

£9.95   0–86242–104–7

CareFully: A guide for home care assistants
Lesley Bell

Recent legislation places increasing emphasis on the delivery of care to older people in their own homes, thereby underlining the crucial role of Home Care Assistants. This accessible guide provides practical advice on the day-to-day tasks encountered and addresses such issues as legal responsibilities and emotional involvement.

£9.95   0–86242–129–2

Reminiscence and Recall: A guide to good practice
Faith Gibson
Reminiscence work is acknowledged as a successful therapy in the care of older people. This new guide provides practical advice on planning and running reminiscence activity in a residential or day care setting and examines suitable approaches for people with particular conditions.
£9.95   0–86242–142–X

The 36-Hour Day: A family guide to caring at home for people with Alzheimer's disease and other confusional illnesses
Nancy L Mace and Peter V Rabins MD
Now in a new edition, this highly successful, sensitive guide carries information on the medical, legal, financial and emotional aspects of caring, combining practical advice with specific examples.
Co-published with Headway.
£9.99   0–34056–382–6

Money Matters

Other People's Money: Guidance on the responsibilities of formal carers in the NHS
Report of Age Concern, MENCAP, MIND, NAHAT and the Disabled Living Foundation
Aims to help formal carers to understand the practical issues involved in designing and putting into practice policies to assist people to manage their own money.
For further information, please contact Donna Pearce on 081-679 8000.

Managing Other People's Money
Penny Letts
Foreword by The Master of The Court of Protection
The management of money and property is usually a personal and private matter. However, there may come a time when someone else has to take over on either a temporary or a permanent basis. This book looks at the circumstances in which such a need could arise and provides a step-by-step guide to the arrangements which have to be made.
£5.95   0–86242–090–3

Your Rights: A guide to money benefits for older people
Sally West

A highly acclaimed annual guide to the State benefits available to older people. Contains current information on income support, housing benefit, council tax benefit and retirement pensions, among other sources of financial help, and includes advice on how to claim them.

For further information, please ring 081-679 8000.

Policy

Financing Long-Term Care
William Laing

Funding long-term care for older people is a major issue which still remains largely unaddressed by politicians. This book sets the subject in its demographic and social context, and explores the economic costs of care in the UK and the experience of other countries. A wide range of policy options are put forward to tackle the problem, including new insurance products.

£14.95   0–86242–123–3

The Law and Vulnerable Elderly People
Edited by Sally Greengross

This report raises fundamental questions about the way society views and treats older people. The proposals put forward seek to enhance the self-determination and autonomy of vulnerable old people while ensuring that those who are physically or mentally frail are better protected in the future.

£6.50   0–86242–050–4

To order books, send a cheque or money order made payable to Age Concern England to the address below. Postage and packing are free. Credit card orders may be made on 081-679 8000.

ACE Books
Age Concern England
PO Box 9
London SW16 4EX

INFORMATION FACTSHEETS

Age Concern England produces over 30 factsheets on a variety of subjects.

To order factsheets

Single copies are available free on receipt of a 9″ × 6″ sae. If you require a selection of factsheets or multiple copies totalling more than five, charges will be given on request.

A complete set of factsheets is available in a ring binder at the current cost of £34, which includes the first year's subscription. The current cost for annual subscription for subsequent years is £15. There are different rates of subscription for people living abroad.

Factsheets are revised and updated throughout the year and membership of the subscription service will ensure that your information is always current.

For further information, or to order factsheets, write to:

Information and Policy Department
Age Concern England
1268 London Road
London SW16 4ER

Index